Forty Days of Care
for the Caregiver

To Marie —
Thanks for caring!
Vicki Gilliam
I Peter 5:7

Forty Days of Care for the Caregiver

Inspirational and Informational Readings
for Those Who Give Care to Others

Dr. Vicki L. Gilliam

Pleasant Word
A Division of WINEPRESS PUBLISHING

ISBN 1-4141-0203-8
Library of Congress Catalog Card Number: 2004093542

Dedication

This book is dedicated to my mother,
Lucille Mabry Gilliam,
who has been both caregiver and
care recipient in my life
and who continues to care for me in
innumerable ways.

Table of Contents

Introduction

"When one is sick . . . two need help."
(The Well Spouse Foundation)

Why write a devotional book of "care" for the caregiver? Consider these recent statistics from the National Family Caregivers Association:

- More than one quarter (26.6%) of the adult population has provided care for a chronically ill, disabled, or aged family member or friend during the past year. Based on 2000 U.S. Census Data, that translates into more than 50 million people.
- Caregiving is no longer predominantly a women's issue. Men now make up 44% of the caregiving population.
- As of 1995, people over 85 years of age are the fastest growing segment of the population. Half of them need some help with personal care.
- Sixty-one percent (61%) of "intense" family caregivers (those providing at least 21 hours of care a week) have suffered from depression. Some

studies have shown that caregiver stress inhibits healing.

- Heavy duty caregivers, especially spousal caregivers, do not get consistent help from other family members. One study has shown that as many as three fourths of these caregivers are "going it alone."
- Approximately 80% of home care services are provided by family caregivers.
- A recent study by Met Life estimates that American businesses lose between $11 billion and $29 billion each year due to employees' need to care for loved ones 50 years of age and older.
- The economic value of services that family caregivers provide "for free" is estimated at $257 billion a year.
- Fifty-nine percent of the adult population either is or expects to be a family caregiver.[1]

In the so-called "graying of America," the median age of the United States population has been rising and is expected to continue to rise well into the mid-twenty-first century. In 1900, one American in twenty-five was age sixty-five or older; in 1984, one in nine. By the middle of this century, it is estimated that one in five Americans will be elderly as the "baby-boom" generation continues to age.[2] Accordingly, eldercare is projected to replace childcare as the number one dependent care issue by 2005.

Senior adults are not the only population that requires caregiving, however. Advances in medicine and medical technology result in people with significant physical and cognitive needs living longer and in greater numbers. More and more, family members are called upon to become caregivers to mentally-challenged adult siblings, loved ones with life-changing injuries, extremely premature babies, and children with significant disabilities. Another trend in current American society finds senior adults caring for relatives under the age of eighteen. For example, according to the 2000 U.S. Census Data, more than two million grandparents have taken on primary responsibility for their grandchildren's basic needs.

Former First Lady Rosalynn Carter summarizes statistics such as these in a thought-provoking manner:

"There are only four kinds of people in this world:
Those who have been caregivers,
Those who currently are caregivers,
Those who will be caregivers, and
Those who will need caregivers."[3]

Obviously, the physical, emotional, and economic implications of these trends are significant. Organizations such as the American Association of Retired Persons (AARP), the National Alliance for Caregiving, the National Family Caregivers Association, the Family Caregiver Alliance, and other private and governmental agencies are reaching out to caregivers to address these needs. However, caregivers also have spiritual needs that may not be addressed so readily. The purpose of this book is to address these spiritual needs while providing helpful and inspirational information to the caregiver.

Who is a caregiver? My favorite definition is from the National Family Caregiver Association: "We are family, friends, and neighbors who stand by those we love as they face chronic illness or disability. We share a common bond with each other despite the fact that some of us care for our spouses, while others care for parents, children or [other loved ones], and despite the fact that we

11

deal with a wide array of medical conditions and diag-noses."[4] For the purpose of this book, the definition can be expanded to include those who provide care for a living. "Professional" caregivers such as nurses, home health care providers, and nursing home or hospice staff may also find inspiration from these devotionals.

Why "forty days" of care? Obviously, forty days do not translate into a week, a month, or any other common group-ing of days; however, Bible students have long considered forty days to be spiritually significant. Remember, Noah was in the flood for 40 days and 40 nights; Moses was on Mount Sinai for 40 days and 40 nights; and Jesus was in the wilder-ness for 40 days and 40 nights—to name a few. In the nu-meric system of the Scriptures, the number "40" consistently is associated with completion and with spiritual prepara-tion.[5] It is my hope that as you complete these forty days of care, you will be more spiritually prepared to realize the joys and to deal with the challenges that come from caregiving.

Why me? A caregiver myself, I decided to write a de-votional book for caregivers after retiring with thirty-one years as an educator. Most of those years were spent work-ing in special education programs for students with dis-abilities and their parents. Professionally, I have experienced first-hand the care and dedication given by parents, loved ones, and teachers to children and teenag-ers with significant disabilities.

In addition to working with individuals with spe-cial needs, I have felt God's call to three other specific things in my life: (1) children's ministries when I was younger, (2) senior adult ministries when I couldn't keep up with the kids anymore, and (3) caring for my mother when advancing age and medical conditions created that need. These areas of my life have given me professional and personal experiences that I have incorporated into these devotionals and that, hopefully, will provide inspiration for others to whom God has entrusted the care of a loved one.

In this book, you will find forty daily devotionals, related Scripture passages, and original poem-prayers. Integrated into these devotionals are facts and tips for caregivers from numerous national and state caregiver resources so that they will be informational as well as inspirational. My prayer is that, as you study these pages, you will find or renew the faith, hope, and love so necessary in the life and heart of a very special person—a caregiver.

"You are quiet heroes, unknown except to your loved one and closest friends."

(Nancy Wexler, gerontologist)

DAY 1

Taking Care of You ...

Caregivers need care, too! We all know it, but we just have a hard time doing it. A recent study by the National Alliance for Caregiving and the AARP found that more than half of those who provide major care for a loved one experience stress and emotional strain. AARP considers this finding a major concern since prolonged stress can lead to significant emotional and physical consequences. As a result, taking care of ourselves is one of the most important aspects of taking care of others effectively.

"Because you're responsible for the welfare of another person, taking care of yourself is doubly important," says the American Heart Association. "You need to stay rested, refreshed and energetic both for yourself and for the person you care for."[1]

PacifiCare offers similar advice: "You, the caregiver, are incredibly important. The welfare of another person depends upon you. If you are not in good health, that other person may also suffer. So, if you've taken on the role of a caregiver, you've also accepted a special responsibility to take care of yourself. That means taking care of yourself physically, emotionally, mentally, spiritually, interpersonally, and financially."[2]

What are some practical ways that we, as caregivers, can take care of ourselves? AARP offers these suggestions: (1) take care of your health, especially nutrition, exercise, and sleep, (2) maintain or establish social contacts to avoid isolation, (3) ask friends and relatives for help with daily tasks and errands, (4) deal constructively with negative feelings, and (5) find time for yourself to unwind and to have fun. Also, avoid bottled-up feelings by talking with family and friends about the rewards and challenges of caregiving and by sharing your experiences with coworkers in similar situations.[3]

Taking care of ourselves physically and emotionally is key, but even more importantly, we must take care of ourselves spiritually. Finding time for prayer, Bible study, worship, and Christian fellowship is vital in the spiritual life of a caregiver. All of these things take time, but they give us the strength to do more with the time that remains. And remember, God's Word gives us a precious promise: God cares for each of us, and because He cares, He desires that we give our frustrations, our concerns, and our cares to Him. Lean on Him. He is the very best Caregiver!

"Cast all your cares on Him because He cares for you."
(1 Peter 5:7)

Help us turn to You, dear Lord,
When things are tough and times are hard.
And every time we shed a tear,
Help us remember you are near.

DAY 2

Wrapping in the Warmth . . .

L ike most of you, I am a caregiver. I have the privilege and the challenge of caring for my mother, who came to live with me about eight years ago when she was eighty years of age. By the time she reached her mid-eighties, my mother had lost her ability to bathe and dress alone due to a series of strokes that affected her motor skills more than her communication or memory. When I first began helping with her bath and drying her afterwards, she seemed to enjoy the baths and appreciate the help, but she was always cold, especially when she first got out of the tub. We tried warmer water, faster baths, and extra heaters, but nothing seemed to get rid of that initial chill.

Then one day, I had an idea. Before her bath, I placed her towel in the clothes dryer to warm, and as she exited the bathtub, I wrapped the warm towel all the way around her upper body in a bearhug fashion. The warm towel dispelled the chill, and the "bear hug" technique basically dried her entire upper body all at once. "Oh, that feels *so* good it makes me want to purr," she exclaimed, and warm towels quickly became a regular part of our bath routine. Especially on cold mornings, wrapping in the warmth of a heated towel protects her from the cold surroundings. (And I don't think she minds the big hug either!)

We are much the same in our spiritual lives. We can grow cold spiritually when the demands of life steal our time to be quiet and still before God. We can feel cold and alone when we are moving too fast to feel the warmth of the Son. We may even find ourselves crying out as David did, "Therefore is my spirit overwhelmed within me; my heart within me is desolate" (Psalm 143:4 KJV).

When the world seems cold and desolate all around you, and when the remedies of this world don't seem to help, allow God to wrap you in the warmth of His love and hold you in the strength of His arms.

"How precious is Your lovingkindness, O God! Therefore the children of men put their trust under the shadow of Your wings."

(Psalm 36:7 HCSB)

Thank you for the love you give
Every moment that we live.
You will keep us safe and warm
In your strong and loving arms.

DAY 3

Being Content...

Caregivers often completely change their lifestyles to take care of those they love.[1] For some Christians, this lifestyle change may involve their public service to the Lord. Consider the following poem by Ruth Harms Calkin:

"I Wonder"

You know, Lord, how I serve You
With great emotional fervor
In the limelight.
You know how eagerly I speak for You
At the women's club.
You know how I effervesce when I promote
A fellowship group.
You know my genuine enthusiasm
At a Bible study.

But how would I react, I wonder,
If You pointed to a basin of water
And asked me to wash the calloused feet
Of a bent and wrinkled old woman
Day after day
Month after month
In a room where nobody saw
And nobody knew.[2]

These words may become an accurate "before-and-after" portrait for Christians who become caregivers. The "what if" of the second verse becomes reality, and years of very public service are replaced with the very private calling of caring for a loved one. With such a change in lifestyle, how do caregivers stay content? In Philippians 4:12, Paul says he has learned the secret of being content in any and every situation. What is Paul's secret of contentment? His answer can be found in the next verse: "I can do *all* things through Christ who strengthens me" [HCSB, EMPHASIS ADDED]. When we seek His purpose in every stage of our lives, Christ will give us strength to do whatever He calls us to do, whether it be in the spotlight or in a room where nobody sees and nobody knows.

". . . for I have learned to be content whatever the circumstances. I know what it is to be in need, and I know what it is to have plenty. I have learned the secret of being content in any and every situation . . ."
(Philippians 4:11b–12a)

Lord, I can serve you on a stage
Or in a room or on a page.
Help me love "the least of these,"
Especially when no one sees.

Looking Good...

ooking good has always been important to my
mother. Let me rephrase that: Looking *great* has always been *very* important to my mother. Twice
weekly visits to the beauty salon for hair and nails had been
a part of her schedule for as long as I can remember. Her
shoes, purse, and jewelry always matched her dress or
pant-suit. In recent years, strokes had robbed her of the
ability to drive and the endurance to shop, but her desire
to look good was as strong as ever. For me, that meant
frequent trips to take her to her hair stylist and her nail
technician, as well as many visits to the mall to shop for
her—none of which were "my thing." They were important to her, though, so I tried to make them important to
me—although not without occasional grumbling!

Then she experienced an illness requiring surgery that
drained her physically and emotionally. Many days
passed without her usual emphasis on looking good. She
would not or could not go to the beauty salon, and she
frequently preferred not to change out of her gown and

robe at all. By the time she had recovered and had begun to show interest in her appearance again, my grumbling had disappeared. (Most of the time!) I had learned an important lesson: How she looked on the outside reflected how she felt on the inside.

Consider this information from the *CareGuide*: "If you look good, you generally feel good, too. Few things raise the spirit like newly coiffed hair and a freshly laundered shirt. . . . As aging fingers lose their flexibility, and as arthritis or other aging-related ailments rob us of our former strength, the simple act of dressing and grooming can prove more and more difficult. Helping your elder look and smell fresh everyday can be a great boost to her self-esteem."[1]

I am reminded of Jesus' anointing at Bethany. The Scriptures tell us that just a few days before His death, a woman came to Jesus with an alabaster jar of very expensive perfume. She broke the jar and poured the perfume on His head. Some of those present criticized her for wasting perfume that could have been sold for money to help the poor. Jesus responded, "Leave her alone. Why are you bothering her? She has done a beautiful thing to me. The poor you will always have with you . . . but you will not always have me." She did *what* she could *while* she could. So should we.

"Whom shall I send, and who will go for us? And I said, Here am I. Send me."

(Isaiah 6:8)

Little things that seem so small
Can be important, after all.
Lord, help me go and get and do
As if I did it all for You.

22

Showing Your Love...

I do a lot of internet shopping for Christmas and birthday gifts, and as a result, I receive a multitude of catalogs. One in today's mail advertised a caregiver coffee mug. On the mug was this reminder: "Take good care every day to show your love in a special way."[1]

How can a caregiver show her love everyday in a special way? To be sure, all the routine tasks of caregiving should demonstrate the caregiver's love, but how can we go above and beyond the routine to show love in *a special way*? Of course, there are tangible things such as cards, flowers, gifts, and such, but sometimes the most important things cost little or no money. Here are a few suggestions:

- Listen to your loved one. Finding time to listen to stories and memories—even if you've heard them more than once—affirms that what he has to say is important.
- Take time with your loved one to enjoy something she enjoys. Too often, I find myself starting a video

for my mother and then moving on to do something else when I know she enjoys the movie more when I watch it with her.

- Don't underestimate the soothing effect of music and the pleasant memories it can bring to mind. Researchers tell us that hearing and responding to music is one of the last things to be lost to aging, injury, or disability. Learn about your loved one's favorite songs and favorite singers, and then find ways for him to hear them. [2]

- Remember that we never outgrow the need for human touch. If you're not a hugger, a gentle squeeze on the shoulder or even applying lotion or aftershave provides a loving touch that not only communicates your affection but also produces a heightened sense of well-being and security. Scientists tell us that appropriate touch even prompts the brain to produce endorphins, the body's natural pain suppressors, leading to a decreased perception of pain.[3]

- And perhaps most importantly, don't let *what* you are doing become more important than the *person* you are doing it for. For example, a home-cooked meal is wonderful, but sometimes buying or fixing something simple so that you will have time to sit and visit with a loved one may be more important and meaningful for both of you.[4]

Take good care every day to show your love in a special way. That was a reminder I needed today. It's interesting how the Lord can speak even through a mail-order catalog!

"Dear friends, let us love one another, for love comes from God. Everyone who loves has been born of God and knows God."

(1 John 4:7)

Help me listen and really hear
And know the things that they hold dear,
So things I do are never more
Important than those I do them for.

Giving and Receiving...

In June, 2002, I was diagnosed with breast cancer. Thankfully, it was very early stage and could be handled with a partial mastectomy and radiation treatments. Surgery was in July, and I was back at work in three days. I assumed the worst was over . . . and then the radiation treatments began. For seven weeks, every day Monday through Friday, I drove to the cancer center first thing in the morning for my treatments, and then went straight to work. By the end of the third week, the radiation had begun to take its toll, and at the end of each workday, I was just drained. As my friends and family became aware, they began to find ways to help. My secretaries found ways to screen calls and keep my work schedule lighter than usual. My best friends took up the slack in caring for my mother. My staff members even worked out a schedule to provide our evening meal three days a week for a couple of months. In other words, for a period of time, I became the "care-*taker*" rather than the "care-*giver*." It was wonderful—except for one thing: I tend to be more comfortable in the role of the giver than the receiver. Although I knew I couldn't have made it without the help, I often felt awkward and uncomfortable accepting it.

Thinking back on that time in my life, I am reminded of Simon Peter. He also had a hard time receiving, especially from Jesus. Consider this case in point: To demonstrate the concept of servanthood, Jesus began to wash the disciples' feet. Peter objected, feeling unworthy to accept what was usually a servant's task from the Lord. Jesus made it very clear that on this particular occasion, He wanted Peter to be on the receiving end.

From childhood, most of us have learned "it is more blessed to give than to receive," and it is! However, there are times in our lives when the Lord intends for us to be on the receiving end, and He brings loving, compassionate people into our lives for that purpose. When we fail to accept their assistance, *both we and they* miss out on a wonderful blessing! In the words of Maya Angelou, "When we give cheerfully and accept gratefully, everyone is blessed."[1]

> *"'No,' said Peter, 'you shall never wash my feet.' Jesus answered, 'Unless I wash you, you have no part with me.' 'Then Lord,' Peter replied, 'not just my feet but my hands and my head as well!'"*
>
> (John 13:8–9)

Lord, help me find a way to give
To someone every day I live,
But show me so that I believe
Sometimes You want me to receive.

Resting and Sleeping...

ave you ever felt like the poet Robert Frost when he wrote, ". . . for I have promises to keep and miles to go before I sleep"? All of us experience days when we have more things to do than hours in the day to do them. We push ourselves long and hard, and then when we finally have a few hours to sleep, we can't or don't! Yet, as Dr. Dan Crawford reminds us in his book *DiscipleShape*, "Not even the greatest athlete can run all the time. Rest is as much a part of fitness as is activity. . . . Sometimes the most crucial thing you can do is sleep."[1]

The Alzheimer's Association identifies "sleeplessness" as one of ten warning signs of caregiver stress. When anxiety about facing another day or what the future holds or a seemingly endless list of concerns robs the caregiver of sleep, exhaustion makes it nearly impossible to complete necessary daily tasks.[2]

Have you ever noticed how the Scriptures address every issue we encounter? Well, sleeplessness is no exception. The psalmist wrote, "Surely I will not enter my house, nor lie on my bed; I will not give sleep to my eyes or slumber to my eyelids, until I find a place for the Lord" (Psalm 132:3–5). As Dr. Crawford states, "Ignoring God at bedtime is a sure path to insomnia. On the other hand, reading God's word and communicating with God at bedtime beats sleeping pills."[3]

In Psalm 4, David also gives us this tip for a good night's sleep: ". . . when you are on your beds, search your hearts and be silent. Offer right sacrifices and trust in the Lord." The concerns of today and the anxieties about tomorrow come into proper perspective when we are quiet before the Lord and trust those things to the One who does not sleep or slumber. Knowing that truth, "when you lie down, you will not be afraid; when you lie down, your sleep will be sweet" (Proverbs 3:24).

"He will not let your foot slip—He who watches over you will not slumber; indeed, He who watches over Israel will neither slumber or sleep."

(Psalm 121:3)

Now I lay me down to sleep,
So, Lord, it's up to You to keep
My loved ones safe from harm and sorrow
Till we greet a new tomorrow.

Finding Companionship...

Pookie the cat came to live with my mother a few months after my father died. Pookie was a stray who just took up residence, first on my mother's porch, then in her house, and then in her heart. They just seemed to adopt each other, which came as a surprise to me since my mom had never been especially interested in pets. I, on the other hand, had long been a "cat person" and was pleased to see the companionship and affection this newfound animal friend supplied. During the seven years my mother lived alone, Pookie provided many happy moments and quickly became the focus of my mother's home. I used to joke that she loved Pookie more than she loved me! Even after she and Pookie came to live with me, this feline family member filled the hours for her when she was home alone. As I write this, my mother is eighty-seven, Pookie is about the same age in cat years, and they are still best friends.

My mother is not alone in finding companionship with animal friends. "Pets are an important form of social contact," says Dr. Alan Beck, director of the Center for Human-Animal Bond at Purdue University. [1] "For older people who may be less mobile and who have few or limited companions, animals provide family and friendship, something to care for and to be recognized by." Studies also show that pets can improve physical health by reducing blood pressure, lowering stress, and aiding relaxation. [2]

Wasn't God thoughtful to give us the gift of pets? Each part of God's creation was made with a purpose, and when you think about it, one of the very first tasks God gave to Adam was to name the animals. God once again showed His care for animals when He instructed Noah to save not only humans, but animals of every kind. Even the new heaven and new earth promised after Christ's return is described with animals, where the "wolf also shall dwell with the lamb, and the leopard shall lie down with the kid . . . and a little child shall lead them" (Isaiah 11:6 KJV). As Cecil F. Alexander expressed so beautifully:

> All things bright and beautiful,
> All creatures great and small,
> All things wise and wonderful,
> The Lord God made them all. [3]

And that even includes dogs—a fact that's sometimes a little hard for us "cat people" to accept!

> *"Praise the Lord from the earth, you great sea creatures and all ocean depths, . . . wild animals and all cattle, small creatures and flying birds. . . . Let everything that has breath praise the Lord."*
> (Psalm 148:7, 10 & Psalm 150:6)

For all these creatures great and small
We thank you, Lord; you made them all.
They show us devotion and loyalty
And love us unconditionally.

32

Overcoming Anger...

E ven the most patient caregiver can find himself battling against anger, which may cause him to lash out at his loved one, which leads to feelings of guilt, which can make him feel angry again. Experts call it the anger-guilt-anger cycle, and it's quite common among caregivers.[1]

"Anger comes in many forms," writes Dee Dee Hunt for the International Scleroderma Network. "Anger that they are thrown into the position of caregiver. Anger at downward changes in their loved one's condition. Anger and frustration at the financial consequences experienced if there is a loss of income and health care costs. Anger at having feelings of anger. Anger that no one seems to notice how overwhelming the caregiver's job can be. Anger at loss of control over the situation."[2]

No matter how much the caregiver loves the care recipient, it's almost impossible never to become angry. What matters is what we do with that anger and how we handle it. Here are a few suggestions to get you through the eye of the storm: (1) Leave the room. Walking away, even for a minute or two, may keep you from doing or saying something you'll regret later. (2) Keep your perspective. Is the situation really worth getting angry about? (3) Laugh. Recognize and appreciate the humor in your day-to-day experiences. (4) Don't beat yourself up. If you slip into anger, find a constructive way to deal with it instead of taking a guilt trip. (5) Monitor the frequency and intensity of your anger. If anger permeates your life, you may need to consider a support group or counseling.[3]

Most importantly, follow Paul's advice in his letter to the Ephesians. Deal with anger sooner rather than later. When your anger spills over to your loved ones, don't let that day end without resolving the issue. Often that means putting aside our pride and saying, "I'm sorry." Even if you don't *feel* sorry for the entire incident right at that moment, you can always find at least one thing for which you can legitimately apologize, thus opening lines of communication. As the song lyrics say, "Love is something you *do*. . .not always something you can *feel.*"[4] It may also mean admitting we were wrong. These things are not easy to do, but they are vital in order to keep anger from mushrooming into bitterness, resentment, and unfortunately in some cases, abusive behaviors. Paul states it very clearly in Ephesians 4: "Get rid of all bitterness, rage and anger, brawling and slander, along with every form of malice." Then he goes on to tell us *how*: "Be kind and compassionate to one another, forgiving each other, just as in Christ God forgave you. Be imitators of God, therefore . . . and live a life of love." If, as an act of obedience, we begin to *do* deeds of kindness, compassion, and love, our *feelings* will soon follow suit. In doing so, we are effectively controlling our anger and inviting God to deal with it.[5]

"In your anger do not sin. Do not let the sun go down while you are still angry, and do not give the devil a foothold."
(Ephesians 4:26)

Lord, it always seems we hurt
The ones we love most true.
Replace our anger with deeds of love
That can only come from You.

Having Patience . . .

Branson, Missouri is one of my mother's favorite places to travel. If you've never been to Branson, let me describe it to you: Just north of the Arkansas-Missouri state line, Branson is nestled in the Ozark Mountains, surrounded by an abundance of beautiful scenery. The town itself seems small until you turn west on Highway 76. Suddenly, you encounter a multitude of hotels, motels, restaurants, shops, and music theaters—lots of music theaters! Being a country music fan, my mother has enjoyed seeing concerts there by the likes of Loretta Lynn, Mel Tillis, Glen Campbell, Roy Clark, Jim Stafford, and her favorite—Gene Watson. In addition to country singers, pop and gospel singers of my generation frequently can be found in Branson. We've seen Bobby Vinton, Andy Williams, Pat and Debbie Boone, the Lennon Sisters, the Osmond Brothers, Dino Kartsanokis, and the Blackwoods—to name a few. And then there's Shoji Tabuchi: Every Branson veteran knows about Shoji and his spectacular theater, where even the restrooms are amazing!

Branson is great fun for music lovers, as well as shoppers and nature lovers. There's just one problem: Branson is home to the "world's longest parking lot." Well, it's not actually a parking lot; it's a highway! You see, at certain times of the day and night when the various shows are about to start or have just ended, more cars spill onto Highway 76 than it can handle. The lanes become overloaded, and the cars, trucks, RV's, and buses inch along at a snail's pace, sometimes coming to a complete halt. The city of Branson has worked hard, building secondary roads and alternate routes in recent years to accommodate the growing number of vehicles, but Branson regulars know that sometime during their visit, they're going to get stuck on Highway 76. You know it; you plan for it; and you just make a point to allow enough time to be patient.

Caregiving can be like that, too. Caregivers learn that there will be times when too many things spill into their lives at one time. You know it; you plan for it; and you make a point to be patient. Easier said than done? Yes, when we try to do it on our own, but remember what Paul said about patience in Galatians 5. Paul identified "patience" as one of the fruit of the Spirit. In other words, when we let Him work in us, the Holy Spirit can produce patience in our lives as Christians. Having patience is hard when we try to manufacture it by ourselves, but when we allow the Holy Spirit to enable and empower us, our lives can be characterized by patience, even when we find ourselves on overload!

> *"Better a patient man than a warrior, a man who controls his temper than one who takes a city."*
> (Proverbs 16:32)

"Lord, give me patience and give it now!"
Too often I may say.
So tie me up and slow me down
When I need time to pray.

Maintaining Dignity...

As we care for loved ones who are chronically ill, disabled, or elderly, one of the most important things we can do is to help maintain their dignity. Let me suggest a few ways—some learned from my own mistakes—to do so:

(1) Talk *to* them, not *about* them or *for* them. When a person has limitations requiring a caregiver, others have a tendency to talk in the third person (him, hers, they, etc.) as if the person were not in the room. When the loved one is present, whether it be at a family gathering, a doctor's appointment, or even in the hospital, it is important to talk in terms of "you" or "yours" rather than "him" or "hers." As much as possible, hear what the loved one has to say first, and then as necessary, the caregiver can give input.

(2) Watch the terminology we use as we provide care. For instance, I prefer not to use the word "diapers." Rather, terms such as "disposable underwear" or a

brand name such as "Depends" sound more age-appropriate for adults.

(3) As much as possible, involve your loved one in decisions that affect him or her. Giving input on something as simple as what to have for supper or as important as a change in living arrangements validates his opinion and gives the loved one a sense of being an important part of the family.

(4) Don't assume your loved one no longer needs privacy. Studies have shown that caregivers often forget their loved ones' need for privacy, especially when their level of care involves significant assistance with personal hygiene and grooming.[1]

As always, Jesus is our example. He consistently treated people with dignity, no matter what their situation. Think about Zaccheus, a tax collector disdained by society, to whom Jesus said, "I must go to your house today." Remember the woman at the well, considered a social outcast among her people but treated with care and dignity by the Lord. Don't forget the man with leprosy who came to Jesus to be healed. While others kept their distance, Jesus reached out and touched the man. Treating others with dignity, compassion, and unconditional love is not a new idea. It was modeled perfectly for us by the One who loved us enough "that while we were yet sinners, He died for us" (Romans 5:8).

"She is clothed with strength and dignity; she can laugh at the days to come."

(Proverbs 31:25)

You never judge what's outside
But always look within.
Help me, Lord, to see what is,
But not forget what's been.

DAY 12

Sharing Laughter...

I am not a morning person! Everyone who knows me well knows that fact to be true. On the other hand, my mother is an early-to-bed-early-to-rise person. She gets up early because she *wants* to; I get up early because I *have* to. As a result, I'm not much of a talker at the breakfast table. Not long after my mother moved in with me, we were having coffee together, and in an off-handed way of expressing my dislike of getting up early that day, I simply muttered, "Bluh!" Laughing, my mother responded with her own version of "bluh," and with those two utterances, we had a pretty good idea of how each of us felt that morning. As the days and weeks passed, our daily "bluhs" became a routine part of our early morning coffee with the frequency, intensity, and volume reflecting how we were feeling that morning. It's our own private joke, and sometimes now we even rank things as being "three-bluh" or "five-bluh," etc., as if we have our own rating scale for life. It's silly, but it's given us something to laugh about, even on mornings when I don't want to be awake or on days when she's not feeling particularly well.

For a long time, *Reader's Digest* has reminded us that "laughter is the best medicine," and there's a great deal of truth in that. In fact, Solomon said it first in Proverbs 17:22: "A cheerful heart is good medicine, but a crushed spirit dries up the bones." The importance of laughter in the life of both the caregiver and the care recipient is well-documented. Even during the Middle Ages, Henri de Mondeville, a professor of surgery, instructed, "Let the surgeon take care to regulate the whole regimen of the patient's life for joy and happiness, allowing his relatives and special friends to cheer him, and by having some one tell him jokes. The surgeon must forbid anger, hatred and sadness in the patient and remind him that the body grows fat from joy and thin from sadness."[1]

Several centuries later, Mark Twain concurred: "The human race has only one really effective weapon, and that's laughter. The moment it arises, all our hardnesses yield, all our irritations and resentments slip away, and a sunny spirit takes their place." More recently, numerous studies have suggested that "there are positive effects to be gained from laughter as a great tension-releaser, pain reducer, breathing improver, and general elevator of moods."[2]

We are "fearfully and wonderfully made," and a part of God's design includes our bodies' physiological and psychological responses to laughter. Laughter does indeed affect the body, mind, and spirit. Thank you, Lord, for the gift of laughter!

"And Sarah said, "God hath made me to laugh, so that all who hear will laugh with me."

(Genesis 21:6 KJV)

Help us see the humor, Lord,
In things you bring our way.
Not laughing at but laughing with
Can brighten all our days.

Accepting Change...

When parents grow older and need progressively increasing care, it is often the adult child who transitions into caregiver. In recent years, expressions such as "role reversal," "parenting the parent," and "parent-child turnabout" have commonly been used to describe this transition. However, some experts on aging have begun to question the use of these terms, as evidenced in this quote from Beverly Pfeiffer:

"The notion that child and parent are "reversing roles" reflects misconceptions about aging and about caregiving. . . . Experts on aging suggest we reframe our thinking about dependence and independence in terms of the acceptance of another stage of development in life, rather than role reversal. This can help caregivers to accept their parent's need for help without treating them as children either in action or tone of voice."[1]

Nevertheless, accepting changes in the parent-child relationship is a part of the caregiving process. "It can be a difficult transition for a child to take on the role of . . .

decision-maker," says Dr. Diana Kerwin of the Medical College of Wisconsin's Division of Geriatrics and Gerontology. The adult child "needs to be empowered to step in and begin caring for their ailing parent—making sure their parent takes his or her medication, for instance, or telling their parent they should not drive, and making difficult decisions about when the parent is no longer able to safely live alone."[2]

So while the roles may not reverse, they do change, and this realization may generate a myriad of emotions in both the aging parent and the adult child. These emotions need to be recognized, acknowledged, and discussed so that the changes can be accepted as another part of God's plan. As Linda Neukrug says in her *Guidepost* prayer, "Dear God, thank You for Your love that follows us throughout our lives. May I never lose my sense of wonder at how wonderfully You bring us from babyhood to adulthood."[3] God is there through all the ages and stages of our lives and the many changes that accompany them. With that knowledge, accepting those changes becomes a matter of faith rather than emotion.

"Surely goodness and mercy shall follow me all the days of my life . . ."

(Psalm 23:6, EMPHASIS ADDED)

"Thou shalt honor . . ." does not cease
Just because we're grown.
May our care be done with thoughtfulness
And reflect the love You've shown.

Holding on Through the Rough Times...

My great-niece Hannah recently took her first air-plane flight. As the plane climbed through the clouds toward cruising altitude, she excitedly told her mom and grandparents, "We're going up to where God is!" As they continued to climb, the plane suddenly encountered unexpected turbulence, at which point Hannah proclaimed, "I think we've already gone past Him!" In her special five-year-old way, she had described her concept of God as a loving heavenly Father who keeps us safe from danger and harm. To her, the safety of being "where God is" did not match the turbulence she was feeling in that airplane.

As Hannah continues to grow, she will come to understand that life consists of both smooth flights and turbulent rides. Thankfully, God is there when things are smooth *and* when things get bumpy. As the Scriptures promise, nothing can separate us from His love.

Some care recipients have conditions, such as Alzheimer's, that may cause them to have good days and bad days. "A person with Alzheimer's can change from day-to-day, hour-to-hour, minute-to-minute. . . . They may be clear headed and cheerful in the morning, but confused, agitated and hostile by lunchtime," according to the Canadian Medical Association.[1] As a result, the caregiver's "ride" can be smooth on one day and turbulent the next. It is a blessing to know that no matter how much turbulence we face, we can never get bumped beyond "where God is." As the psalmist wrote, "If I go up to the heavens, you are there; if I make my bed in the depths, you are there. If I rise on the wings of the dawn, if I settle on the far side of the sea, even there your hand will guide me, your right hand will hold me fast" (Psalm 139:8–10). When things are smooth, don't forget to thank Him for His constant presence, but when things get bumpy, don't hesitate to hang on tight to His strong and loving hand!

"For I am convinced that neither death nor life, neither angels nor demons, neither the present nor the future, nor any powers, neither height nor depth, nor anything else in all creation, will be able to separate us from the love of God that is in Christ Jesus our Lord."

(Romans 8:38–39)

Thank you for the good times,
And thanks when things get rough.
It's then You hold us tighter,
So we know Your strength's enough.

Being Satisfied, Not "Sandwiched"...

In the world of caregiving, there is a distinct group sometimes referred to as the "sandwich generation." These are mostly baby boomers between the age of forty-five and fifty-five who are caring for both their parents and their children. Since this term was coined by Carol Abaya, much has been written about the pressures of managing both children and aging parents and the various techniques used to cope with the stress of being "in the middle."

Recently, AARP conducted a national study of this population to learn their characteristics, feelings, and coping mechanisms, and received rather unexpected responses from the so-called "Me Generation."

"The results of the study are intriguing, and even surprising," AARP reports. "They show a generation who tell us that family is the most important thing in their lives. Respondents said they welcome the opportunity to be involved in the care of their loved ones. . . . They are generally comfortable with their family roles, and self-confident as they manage the dual responsibilities of parents and children." [1] In other words, these caregivers are feeling *satisfied* rather than *sandwiched*.

Perhaps AARP found these results somewhat surprising because feelings of satisfaction can be elusive—both in our emotional and our spiritual selves. We might call it the "Grass-Is-Always-Greener Syndrome." Nevertheless, the Bible gives us guidance on how to become and remain spiritually satisfied. Here are some of those whom God has promised in His Word to satisfy:

1. *The meek who seek*—"The meek shall eat and be *satisfied*: they shall praise the Lord that seek him . . ." (Psalm 22:26 KJV, EMPHASIS ADDED).

2. *The just who trust*—"How excellent is thy lovingkindness, O God! therefore the children of men put their trust under the shadow of thy wings. They shall be abundantly *satisfied* . . ." (Psalm 36:7–8 KJV, EMPHASIS ADDED).

3. *Those who praise all their days*—"Thus will I bless thee while I live: I will lift up my hands in thy name. My soul shall be *satisfied* as with marrow and fatness; and my mouth shall praise thee with joyful lips" (Psalm 63:4–5 KJV, EMPHASIS ADDED); "*Satisfy* us in the morning with your unfailing love, that we may sing for joy and be glad all our days" (Psalm 90:14 EMPHASIS ADDED).

4. *Those who call when they fall*—"Because he loves me, says the Lord, I will rescue him; I will protect him, for he acknowledges my name. He will call upon me, and I will answer him; I will be with him in trouble, I will deliver him and honor him. With long life will I *satisfy* him and show him my salvation" (Psalm 91:14–16 EMPHASIS ADDED).

"The fear of the Lord tendeth to life; and he that hath it shall abide <u>satisfied</u>; he shall not be visited with evil."

(Proverbs 19:23 KJV, EMPHASIS ADDED)

Lord, You know I'm satisfied
With all You did and how You died
From sin and shame to set us free!
But are you satisfied with me?

Putting on the Armor...

My great-nephew Zachary is learning to play ice hockey. During the first dozen or so lessons, the only equipment required was his helmet. Once he reached "Hockey 3" lessons, however, he was required to wear full gear. As I helped him locate, purchase, and put on the equipment for the first time, I gained a new appreciation for hockey players. They wear a *lot* of stuff under those uniforms. There are the shoulder pads, which protect not only the shoulders, but also the chest and upper back. There are thick padded pants, elbow pads, shin guards, a neck cover and, for lack of a better term, a hockey jockey. Add to all of that a pair of thick padded gloves, ankle-to-knee socks, the helmet with a metal face cage, and the ice skates, and only *then* is the hockey player ready to pick up his offensive weapon—the hockey stick. Especially in youth hockey, the players must prepare themselves in all the appropriate protective gear before they can ever take their stand on the ice.

In a spiritual sense, God instructs Christians to do something very similar. In Ephesians 6, Paul tells us to put on the full armor of God so that we can take our stand against Satan's schemes, and then he specifies the pieces of armor— our spiritual "equipment"—to put on. Notice the order: first, the belt of *truth,* the breastplate of *righteousness,* the "shoes" of *readiness,* the shield of *faith,* and the helmet of *salvation.* Then, after we have prepared ourselves with our "protective gear," we are to take up the only offensive weapon Paul mentions—"the sword of the Spirit, which is the *word of God"* [EMPHASIS ADDED]. As Christians, we must prepare ourselves in all the appropriate spiritual armor so that when the devil attacks, we will be able to "stand our ground" and "extinguish all the flaming arrows of the evil one."

For us as caregivers, what are some of the "flaming arrows" the evil one may decide to throw our way? In the words of the Alzheimer's Association, here are a few: Depression ("I just don't care anymore"), anxiety ("What happens when he needs more care than I can give?"), anger ("If she asks me that same question one more time, I'll scream!"), social withdrawal ("I just don't have the energy to get together with our neighbors anymore"), and health problems ("I can't remember the last time I felt good").[1] Thankfully, Paul assures us that we can extinguish these flaming arrows with the shield of faith, and we can fight back with our spiritual sword, which is the Word of God.

> *"Be strong in the Lord and in His mighty power. Put on the full armor of God so that you can take your stand against the devil's schemes."*
>
> (Ephesians 6:10–11)

The devil is an evil coward
Seeking whom he may devour,
So help me keep my armor ready,
Shield held high, and sword held steady.

Saying "No"...

Saying "no" can be one of the most difficult tasks for a caregiver, especially when the care recipient is a parent. Brenda Jones Vieregg, one of the authors of *Fourteen Friends' Guide to Eldercaring*, identified part of the problem in this way: "The reason eldercaring is so difficult is that, besides the physical work which we all can do when you're caring for somebody, it involves the longest relationship of our whole life. And so you bring all of the emotions of that relationship into the caring process."[1] Yet, setting limits by saying "no" is sometimes necessary in the caregiving relationship for at least two reasons. First, saying "no" is vital when it's in the best interest of the loved one receiving care. Illness, disability, or the aging process may cause the care recipient to have unrealistic expectations or the desire to participate in activities that are no longer appropriate. A common example is driving after it is no longer safe for the loved one to do so. Even though it's difficult, the adult child, adult sibling, or caregiving spouse needs to say "no" for the safety and well-being of the care recipient as well as others.

Additionally, setting limits by saying "no" is sometimes necessary for the physical and emotional well-being of the caregiver. Finding a balance in taking care of your loved one and taking care of yourself can be tricky. "Your care receiver may need constant reassurance about his/her safety, your love, medical care or costs, changes in your life together . . . or any other number of personal concerns. Your ability to listen to their concerns is very important," caregiving experts advise. On the other hand, "all caregivers should receive respite regularly. Give yourself permission to ask for help. Turn to other people for help—your family, friends, church/synagogue, and neighbors. Allow yourself a break from your caregiving responsibilities."[2] Accomplishing this may mean saying "no"—even to a parent—without feeling guilty.

Perhaps it will help to remember that even our loving heavenly Father sometimes says "no" to our requests. Unlimited by time and space, our omniscient, omnipresent God sees the big picture, and because of His unconditional love, He acts in our best interest by sometimes saying "no" or "wait" or "not right now" to our prayers.

Therein lies the secret to saying "no" appropriately as a caregiver: look at the big picture, decide what's in the best interest of those involved, and act with unconditional love.

"Going a little farther, he fell with his face to the ground and prayed, 'My Father, if it is possible, may this cup be taken from me. Yet not as I will, but as you will.'"
(Matthew 26:39)

"Take this cup if it be Your will,"
In agony Christ prayed.
Help us accept the "no's" as well
As He did on that day.

Finding Beauty . . .

Today's devotional consists of the words to a song I wrote several years ago. They will probably be most meaningful to those who are caregivers for children with disabilities, but I believe there is meaning to be found by any caregiver.

Butterflies and Rainbows

Said the caterpillar to the lovely butterfly,
"Why aren't you ugly like me?
You have beautiful colors, you can
soar in the sky
And I can only crawl on this tree."
But the butterfly replied, "Keep on
climbing that tree.
Keep working and doing your best.
Keep reaching for the sky, my friend,
and you will see
Time will take care of the rest."

Said the dark, rainy cloud to the bright sunshine,
"Why aren't you ugly like me?
You can brighten up the world; you
can make it fine,
And I can only cry constantly."
But the sunshine replied, "Come along with me.
We'll work together wherever we go.
Add your sparkle to my glowing, friend,
and you will see.
We'll paint the skies with lovely rainbows."

Said that special child to others all around,
"Why aren't you ugly like me?
You can learn; you can walk;
and it gets me down . . .
All the things I can't do easily."
But a friend reaches out her hand and
says with a smile,
"Let me show you all the things you can do.
Keep reaching for the sky, my friend,
and in a while,
We'll find the butterflies and
rainbows in you."

"He has made everything beautiful in its time. He has
also set eternity in the hearts of men; yet they cannot
fathom what God has done from beginning to end."
(Ecclesiastes 3:11)

Help me see the butterflies
And not the old cocoon.
Help me find the rainbows, Lord,
For they are gone so soon.

Putting the Pieces Together...

Between the time my father retired in 1979 and went to be with the Lord in 1988, he completed a large number of jigsaw puzzles. Not being one to just sit and watch TV, he always seemed to have a puzzle going on a card table in the den. We didn't realize how many though until after his death, when we found a large stack of puzzles separated by poster board under his bed. Recently, therefore, hearing a luncheon speaker use a jigsaw puzzle analogy reminded me of my dad . . . not just because of the puzzles themselves, but also the lessons learned from them.[1] I decided that "lessons from a jigsaw puzzle" had something to say to caregivers, as well.

1. *Establish the border first.* In puzzles and in caregiving, boundaries are necessary and important.
2. *Don't force a fit.* Forcing someone or something to fit where it doesn't belong may be a temporary solution but will usually cause problems in the long run.

3. *Look at the big picture* and don't get bogged down with the little pieces. It's easy sometimes to lose sight of the forest for the trees.

4. *When nothing seems to come together, take a break.* Things often look different when you come back to them.

5. *Doing it right takes time.* Putting all the pieces together correctly can be a lengthy process. Don't rush or become impatient.

6. *Pieces can fall apart without the proper glue.* To avoid falling to pieces, depend on the "glue" that holds our lives together . . . friends "who *stick* closer than a brother" and the special Friend we have in Jesus (Proverbs 18:24 EMPHASIS ADDED).

7. *Follow the guide given by the creator.* The creator of a puzzle provides a picture of the finished product to use as a guide. Our Creator also provides a Guide to follow for those "who receive the word with all readiness of mind, and search the scriptures daily" (Acts 17:11 KJV).

8. *One missing piece makes a difference.* It takes all the pieces to complete the picture. The proverb says, "It takes the whole village to raise a child." In like manner, caregiving often needs to be a team effort by family, friends, church, and community.

"And when she hath found it she calleth her friends and her neighbours together, saying, Rejoice with me; for I have found the piece which I had lost."

(Luke 15:9 KJV)

We juggle all the pieces, Lord,
And try to make them fit.
Help us see the big design,
Press on, and never quit.

Encouraging Independence...

Very early in my work with special-needs students, I encountered the term "learned helplessness." I grasped the meaning when my supervisor pointed out to me that in my eagerness to assist students, I was doing *too much* for them. I was doing things they could do, or at least could learn to do, because I was uncomfortable watching them having to work so hard or struggle with a skill. My supervisor wisely helped me realize that in these instances, I was actually doing a disservice rather than helping because the struggle was a part of the learning process. By doing too much, I was teaching the students to depend on others rather than gaining independence.

The same concept comes into play in rehabilitation after illness or injury. Have you ever watched a physical therapist or an occupational therapist as they work with their patients? As family members, we often want to *do for the patient*, but the therapists' approach is to provide treatment and accommodations so that the *patient can do for himself.*

Why? So that the patient can regain or maintain the highest level of independence possible for as long as possible.

Caregivers need to keep the concept of "learned helplessness" in mind as we seek to find a balance between undercare and overcare. When we provide support and empathy instead of over-involvement, we encourage our loved ones to maintain as much independence as they can for as long as possible.

Just the opposite is true, however, in our walk with the Lord. Learning to be dependent on Him is one of the most important aspects of our spiritual growth. The more we try to do on our own, the more likely we are to experience frustration, confusion, and failure. The more we submit to His will and depend on Him for direction, the more likely we are to experience peace, assurance, and blessings in our lives. In Psalm 62, David wrote, "My salvation and my honor depend on God. He is my mighty rock, my refuge. Trust in him at all times, O people; pour out your hearts to him, for God is our refuge." We are helpless without Him, but when we stand "empty-handed before God in total dependence and self-surrender," we find our strength.[1]

"Trust in the Lord with all your heart, and lean not to your own understanding. In all your ways acknowledge him, and he will make your paths straight."

(Proverbs 3:5–6)

Lord, independence is a need
Our human nature seeks.
Help me surrender "self" to You,
For You have blessed the meek.

Evaluating Yourself...

What kind of caregiver are you? What is your caregiving style? Is yours a healthy caregiving relationship? The Caregiver's Self-Rating Scale from the San Diego Mental Health Services is a ten-point continuum which describes the various styles of caregiving, ranging from abandonment to fusion of personalities (see Appendix A). Caregivers can place themselves on the scale to determine how they value the care receiver and how they value themselves.

Take a moment to review the Scale on pages 127–128, and place yourself on the continuum based on the description that sounds most like you. Hopefully, you've identified yourself somewhere in the middle. The low numbers give little or no value to the care receiver, while the high numbers give little or no value to your own needs as an individual. Neither extreme is healthy in the caregiving relationship. Finding yourself at either end of the continuum may be an indication that you need to take action through a support group or counselor.

The Self-Rating Scale is a simple yet meaningful way to evaluate ourselves as caregivers, but how should we evaluate ourselves as Christians? In the first chapter of 2 Peter, there's a simple yet meaningful way to evaluate our spiritual growth. Simon Peter tells us that our goal is to "participate in the divine nature,"—to be like Jesus. Then he gives us a "checklist" of sorts: "Make every effort to add to your *faith, goodness*; and to goodness, *knowledge*; and to knowledge, *self-control*; and to self-control, *perseverance*; and to perseverance, *godliness*; and to godliness, *brotherly kindness*; and to brotherly kindness, *love*. For if you possess these qualities *in increasing measure*, they will keep you from being ineffective and unproductive in your knowledge of our Lord Jesus Christ" (2 Peter 1:5–8 EMPHASIS ADDED). There it is . . . an eight-point "checklist" to evaluate our effectiveness and productivity as we seek to become more and more like Him.

Which of these qualities do you possess? Are you experiencing them "in increasing measure?" Which do you need to add through His divine power?

Are you, as Paul is in 2 Corinthians 3:18, "being transformed into his likeness with ever-increasing glory, which comes from the Lord, who is the Spirit"?

"Examine yourselves to see whether you are in the faith; test yourselves. Do you not realize that Christ Jesus is in you—unless, of course, you fail the test?"
(2 Corinthians 13:5)

We've heard that we're the only Bible
Some will ever read.
Lord, make us more like You so they
Can find the Word they need.

DAY 22

Using Words
Constructively...

For many years, my summers included several Christian children's camps, where I generally led music and fun time. One of the campers' perennial favorites went like this:

> I've got this tongue I can't control.
> It's a fight that I can't win.
> I've got this tongue I can't control,
> And it leads me into sin.
> So I give it to you, my Lord.
> Help it laugh and sing and pray,
> And may it never, never, never, ever
> Stick out at my brother.
> That's my gift to You today![1]

What made this song especially enjoyable for the campers were the sound effects made by wagging the tongue between lines. We had a lot of fun with the song, but it also reminded campers and adult sponsors how easy it is to use the tongue—God's gift of speech—in a hurtful way. It was a lesson we all could use, especially after spending a week together in close communion during the 100+ degree Texas heat.

Of course, this little song was a playful way of teaching the serious lesson we find in the third chapter of James. He compares the tongue to the bit in a horse's mouth, the rudder of a ship, and the spark that starts a forest fire—small items that can cause big things to happen. James reminds us that while humans have tamed almost every animal, we have not been successful taming the tongue. He decries the fact that we praise God and curse God's creation with the same tongue.

Let's think about how this lesson applies to the caregiving relationship in both positive and negative ways. First the negative: Harsh or angry words, criticism, and any communication that puts down rather than lifts up need to be avoided by the caregiver. It's easy to become impatient and say something that we really don't mean or that we will regret later. Caregivers need to be tuned in to this possibility and be careful to put the brain in gear before we put the mouth in motion.

Now, the positive: Our little song makes three good suggestions—laugh, sing, and pray. We have already discussed the importance of laughter and music in previous daily readings, but this will serve as a reminder. Praying with or for the care recipient is another excellent way to use the gift of speech in a positive manner. Reading to the care receiver can help keep communication and thinking skills functioning better and longer. I recently read a review of a book on eldercare, and the reviewer made the observation that while the book had many good suggestions, it completely omitted any reference to reading the Bible. Reading the Bible and singing the "old hymns" to aging loved ones often can be soothing and reassuring.

Finally, make opportunities to use words to build people up, strengthen self-esteem, and acknowledge their accomplishments by implementing an old rule-of-thumb used by teachers . . . give at least four positives for every negative. Then you are using your words constructively, as the Lord intended.

"Do not let any unwholesome talk come out of your mouths, but only what is helpful for building others up according to their needs, that it may benefit those who listen."

(Ephesians 4:29)

Help me laugh and sing and pray
With all the words I use today.
Help me build up and not put down
Every time I make a sound.

Recharging Your Batteries...

You board an airplane and settle into your seat. As the plane leaves the gate, the flight attendant begins to recite the safety instructions given at the beginning of every flight. "In the unlikely event that our cabin loses pressure, an oxygen mask will drop in front of you," the flight attendant demonstrates. "If you are traveling with a child or another person who needs assistance, secure your own mask first, and then help the one who needs assistance." At first blush, that particular instruction may sound selfish or even foolish. After all, a parent's natural reaction in a crisis is to come to the aid of her child first, even if that means putting herself in danger. Upon further reflection, however, the instructions make perfect sense. We are not being told to take care of our own needs *instead of* another's. Rather, the airlines are reminding us to take care of ourselves first so that *we will be able* to take care of others.

That is a reminder that we need as caregivers, as well. Caregivers must give themselves permission to nurture themselves without guilt and with as much compassion as they reserve for others. "Figure out what *your* needs are," urges Professor Alice Domar of the Harvard Medical School. "Then figure out how others in your life can help you meet each need. Each morning, think about something you might do for yourself that day. Remember: If you don't care for yourself, you're less able to care for others."[1]

Even Jesus found it necessary to withdraw from the pressing crowds on occasion. In Luke 5, we are told that after teaching the people "who pressed upon him to hear the word of God," after performing miracles and calling disciples, and after healing many sicknesses, Jesus "withdrew himself into the wilderness, and prayed" (Luke 5:16 KJV). In today's vernacular, Jesus needed time to "recharge His spiritual batteries" after ministering to the multitudes. Jesus was God, but He was God in a human body that needed physical, emotional, and spiritual renewal at times. Why should we feel inadequate when we experience the same kind of needs? Find ways to "recharge your batteries," and then find time to do those things. Remember: A "dead battery" doesn't do anybody much good, but a fully-charged battery can keep going and going and going . . .!

"The apostles gathered around Jesus and reported to him all they had done and taught. Then, because so many people were coming and going that they did not even have a chance to eat, he said to them, 'Come with me by yourselves to a quiet place and get some rest.' So they went away by themselves in a boat to a solitary place."

(Mark 6:30–32)

Lord, take me to a quiet place
To be alone with You.
Renew my heart and soul and mind
And give me strength anew.

Working Together for Good...

Where were you on September 11, 2001? What were you doing on November 22, 1963? If you are old enough to remember, who were you with on December 7, 1941? Some dates are indelibly stamped into our memories by tragedies such as the 9/11 attacks, the Kennedy assassination, and Pearl Harbor. For my home church, Wedgwood Baptist in Fort Worth, September 15, 1999, is such a date. On that evening, a disturbed gunman walked into a "See You After the Pole" youth meeting and began firing. Fourteen people were shot, seven died, and many more were traumatized before the shooter turned his gun on himself. It was a dark night for our church family. I remember sleep did not come easily for me that night after learning a choir friend had been killed, a friend from work had been wounded, and another co-worker had lost her daughter. When I awoke early the next morning, I immediately turned on the television, and the local stations were interviewing our pastor, Dr. Al Meredith. As the sun rose over the scene of such darkness, I remember Brother Al quoting Scripture as a part of his response to the media, stating that while our hearts were heavy with sorrow, we would not "grieve like the rest of men, who have no hope." (1 Thessalonians 4:13) Proclaiming "we will not let the powers of darkness overcome the power of light," he was able to witness to the television audience as he continued to respond to the reporters' questions. The local audience became a national audience as he appeared on network news and programs such as Larry King's. But this was only the beginning of God's fulfillment of His promise in Romans 8:28: "And we know that in all things God works for the good of those who love him, who have been called according to his purpose." It would take a book to record all the ways the Lord used people involved in this tragedy to lead others to salvation and to minister to people literally throughout the world. Perhaps Campus Crusade for Christ founder Dr. Bill Bright said it best: "Only God can turn a tearful tragedy into a glorious victory."[1]

Caregiving frequently begins with a tragedy—an unwelcomed diagnosis, a life-altering injury, a grim prognosis, or even the death of a previous caregiver. How should Christian caregivers respond to these tragedies? Author Verdell Davis offers this suggestion: "Most often we cannot choose what happens to us—our choice lies in what we do with what life brings our way. . . .The pains, the heartaches, the losses of our lives can become the altar on which we offer up to God all the things that keep us relying on our own strength. It is then that God can truly do a new work in us and show us Himself in ways we have never seen before."[2]

In his second letter to the Corinthians, Paul stated it this way: "But the Lord said to me, 'My grace is sufficient for you, for my power is made perfect in weakness.' Therefore I will boast all the more gladly about my weaknesses so that Christ's power may rest on me" (2 Corinthians 12:9–10). Only through the power of Jesus Christ can we experience hope and victory in the midst of tragedy. With Him, "weeping may endure for a night, but joy cometh in the morning" (Psalm 30:5 KJV).

"God is our refuge and strength, an ever-present help in trouble. Therefore we will not fear . . ."

(Psalm 46:1–2a)

The night is darkest just before dawn,
But soon we see the Light has come
Rejoicing begins and weeping is gone
When You're the One we lean upon.

Staying Put...

Aging in place is a relatively new term used to describe the trend of continuing to live in the community as independently as possible. According to the Blue Cross and Blue Shield of Texas *LifeTimes* publication, this phenomenon has become so prevalent that designers and builders have begun not only to take notice, but also to take action. In fact, the National Association of Home Builders (NAHB) now offers a three-day certification course for members who want to increase their knowledge of "barrier-free" living environments, as well as the design implications of aging.[1]

Certified Aging in Place Specialists are trained to look ahead to difficulties each of us might encounter as we age so that homes and apartments can be built or remodeled to meet those needs. Their recommendations frequently include such elements as (1) hallways and doors wide enough to accommodate wheelchairs, (2) low-rise thresholds, (3) kitchen counter heights that allow for sitting down while working, (4) non-slip flooring or low density carpet, (5) at least one downstairs bedroom and bath, (6) easy-to-reach and easy-to-read thermostats, and (7) bathrooms prepared for the easy addition of grab bars when needed.

"As we get older, most of us would prefer to be at home where things are familiar," states Mary Jo Peterson, president of a Connecticut consulting firm that specializes in barrier-free design.[2] Now, more than ever, designers and builders can make it not just possible, but easy to age in place . . . to stay put as we mature.

Maturing as a Christian sometimes involves staying put, as well. While we are frequently instructed in the Scriptures to "go," we are sometimes called upon to "wait." Perhaps the best known of these verses is Isaiah 40:31 (KJV): "But they that wait upon the Lord shall renew their strength; they shall mount up with wings as eagles; they shall run, and not be weary; and they shall walk, and not faint."

Why are we sometimes called upon to wait during our Christian walk? I am reminded of my days in high school and college marching bands. As a half-time performance unfolded, our task was usually to move down the field— eight steps for every five yards, in time with the music. Sometimes, however, the band director would instruct some of us to "march in place" so that our legs were moving, but we weren't going anywhere. Why? We were part of his bigger plan, and while we marched in place, the movement all around us would eventually converge into a design or a word that was clear to those watching in the stands. Then, when the time was right, we would move on to the next element in the program.

"Marching in place" as Christians is sometimes necessary so that the Lord can work all around us to make clear His bigger plan. Then in the "fullness of time," He will reveal to us when we should move forward and what our next step should be. In the meantime, He will use that wait-time to renew our strength so that when He says "go," we will be ready to "run and not be weary."

> "Wait on the Lord: be of good courage, and he shall strengthen thine heart: wait, I say, on the Lord."
>
> (Psalm 27:14 KJV)

May we always walk with You
Because we know Your steps are true.
Help us walk the way You've said,
Not lag behind or run ahead.

Walking Toward the Light...

As a young adult, I served as the youth director for several churches in central Texas. Since our youth activities often lasted longer than other church activities, I sometimes found myself turning off lights and locking up the church building after everyone else had gone. At one church, I dreaded a particular hallway on those occasions because of the location of the light switch. Turning the light on when arriving or turning it off when leaving required a trek down the dark hall while it was illuminated only by a small emergency light. When entering to turn on the light, I walked toward the emergency light and could see where I was going and what I was doing. However, after switching it off and turning to leave, I was no longer facing the emergency light, and the same hallway seemed dark and potentially hazardous. What made the difference? It was whether or not I was *walking toward the light*.

Someone has said that placing our faith in the Lord is like driving at night with headlights. An automobile's lights give just enough illumination to drive a certain distance down the road. The driver cannot see beyond that point, but must drive to the edge of the darkness to project more light. This same concept is captured in Proverbs 119:105, where God's Word is described as a "lamp unto my feet," not a spotlight to the far end of the road. When we walk toward the Light with faith, He will always light our path enough to see what our next step should be.

Caregiving is often characterized by uncertainties. What does the future hold? Am I making the right decisions for my loved one? Can I do this alone? For how long? Will our finances hold out? Should we stay here or move? How will my decisions affect other family members? And the list of questions goes on and on . . .

As we face the uncertainties that accompany caregiving, walking toward the Light becomes especially important. I'm reminded of the old gospel song that says,

> Many things about tomorrow
> I don't seem to understand,
> But I know Who holds the future
> And I know Who holds my hand.[1]

When the future seems uncertain, remember that the One who holds the future firmly in His hands stands ready to guide each step we take. When we walk toward the Light and grasp His hand in faith, He will "show us the path of life" . . . one step at a time (Psalm 16:11).

"I will praise the Lord, who counsels me; even at night my heart instructs me. . . . You have made known to me the path of life; you will fill me with joy in your presence, with eternal pleasures at your right hand."

(Psalm 16:7, 11)

We want to know the long-term
While You're showing us the short.
Help us know You see the whole
While we only see in part.

80

Carrying On...

f you're a baby boomer as I am, you will remember a song from the 1970's entitled "He Ain't Heavy; He's My Brother." The lyrics go something like this:

> "The road is long with many a winding turn
> That leads us to who knows where, who knows where,
> But I'm strong, strong enough to carry him.
> He ain't heavy; he's my brother . . .
> So on we go. His welfare is of my concern.
> No burden is he to bear. We'll get there.
> And the load doesn't weigh me down at all.
> He ain't heavy; he's my brother."[1]

For those who have an adult sibling with developmental disabilities or chronic illness, these lyrics may bring mixed feelings. Research indicates that siblings are an integral part of the lives of disabled adults. At the same time, these adult siblings report that one of their greatest concerns is about the future when their parents are no longer able to provide care and support for the brother or sister with special needs, and the weight of responsibility falls on them. While adult siblings consistently report love and concern for the welfare of their disabled brother or sister, believing that "the load doesn't weigh me down at all" may be unrealistic. Trying to mesh their own personal and professional lives with the care of disabled siblings can be difficult. As a result, organizations such as the Arc (a national organization on mental retardation) offer support groups and educational programs for adult siblings who carry or will soon carry the full responsibility of care.[2]

When looking to the Bible for direction in the area of sibling care, the story of Moses comes to mind. Moses depended on his siblings many times throughout his life, so what can we learn from them? Let me suggest at least four things:

First, have a plan and work the plan. As a part of the plan to save his life, Moses' sister Miriam watched out for his safety as a baby in a basket. Miriam worked the plan so well that she even convinced Pharoah's daughter to designate Moses' mother as his nursemaid.

Second, find ways to help and to build the confidence of the disabled sibling at the same time. Brother Aaron became Moses' spokesman when Moses lacked confidence about his own eloquence, but he never took over Moses' appointed role. He did what Moses needed him to do, but he let Moses take the lead.

Third, support the sibling, but don't try to do it all alone. When victory over the Amalekites required Moses to keep his arms lifted all day, Aaron supported his arms when they became tired. Since the task was more than one person could do, Aaron had Hur to help him support Moses' arms until the victory was secure.

Finally, remember these words of wisdom I encountered recently: "Hang in there. Even Moses was once a basket case!"

"A friend loves at all times, and a brother is born for a difficult time."

(Proverbs 17:17 HCSB)

Am I my brother's keeper?
Sometimes the answer's "sure."
Andrew brought his brother;
What have you done for yours?

Working Behind the Scenes...

enjoy the spiritual tidbits frequently found on church signs. Recently as I drove by a church near my home, I noticed these words: "Faith knows that God is working behind the scenes." As I mulled over its meaning, I found two great truths in this saying. First, I focused on the words "faith *knows*." They reminded me that genuine faith does not *think* or *hope* or *wish* or *wonder*. Real faith *knows*. The saying would carry a very different meaning if it read, "Faith hopes that God is working behind the scenes." We don't have to wish or wonder; we simply have to stand on the promises of God. As Paul wrote, "Faith is being *sure* of what we hope for and *certain* of what we do not see" (Hebrews 11:1 EMPHASIS ADDED).

Second, I focused on the phrase "God is working behind the scenes." When I was in high school, I worked as stage manager for several school plays. Working backstage, I quickly realized that what the audience sees on stage is only a small part of a theatrical production. Much goes on behind the scenes to make the production come together as the director envisions it. The same is true on the stage of life. Even when we cannot see obvious manifestations of God's hand in our circumstances, He is still there and involved and working in us "to will and to act according to his good purpose" (Philippians 2:13). God often works in ways we cannot see!

It's comforting to know that we have a God who is working behind the scenes, when so much about caregiving also involves working behind the scenes. In writing about caregivers, gerontologist Nancy Wexler states, "You are quiet heroes, unknown except to your loved one and closest friends."[1] Her statement is correct but incomplete. Caregivers do tend to have vast responsibilities known only to those closest to them, and most often they choose to carry out those responsibilities without compensation, recognition, or tangible reward. To complete Ms. Wexler's statement, however, two words need to be added: "You are quiet heroes, unknown except to your loved one and closest friends *and God.*" God, who works behind the scenes in response to our faith, sees and knows and cares about every good work done in love during the private moments of caregiving.

> *"And if anyone gives even a cup of cold water to one of these little ones because he is my disciple, I tell you the truth, he will certainly not lose his reward."*
>
> (Matthew 10:42)

When we can't see You anywhere,
Give us faith to know You're there
Working in Your way and time
Instead of fitting into mine.

Caring in Sickness and in Health...

*I*n sickness and in health . . . till death do us part. Tradition-
ally, this phrase is spoken by couples as they are joined
in marriage. When life brings chronic illness or disability to one spouse, these words take on new meaning as the
"well spouse" transitions into the role of caregiver.[1] While
the care recipient remains a spouse, he or she may no longer
be able to function as a true life partner, and the well spouse
may grieve the loss of the way the relationship used to be.[2]

Many spousal caregivers report feeling "aloneness," an
emotion distinctly different from loneliness. "Aloneness" is
often a result of the drastic change from having a life partner
with whom to enjoy everyday activities and special events,
to suddenly being thrust into a position of doing things
alone.[3] Others indicate they experience a loss of identity as
the tasks that define the roles in a marriage change.

Decision-making is another area affected by spousal
caregiving. Depending on the loved one's condition,
making decisions about everyday things may change from
a joint effort to an individual one. Spousal caregivers say

that even more troubling are major life decisions which eventually must be made, ranging from when to move to an assisted care facility to whether to approve extensive medical procedures.

For older adults, spousal caregiving can even become a health issue for the caregiver. The Family Caregiver Alliance estimates that spousal caregivers above the age of sixty-five who are experiencing mental or emotional strain have a 63 percent higher risk of dying than non-caregivers in the same age group.[4]

So, with so many issues to deal with, how is a spousal caregiver supposed to cope? Perhaps some of the words to a song I wrote years ago for the wedding of two special friends may offer a few reminders:

> Join our lives, Father, as one.
> Help us hold to one another through Jesus Christ, the Son.
> Give us strength to bear the sorrows with the joys of our tomorrows.
> May we grow to love each other more each day.

> Join our hearts, Father, as we
> Pledge ourselves to one another to love eternally.
> Bind our hearts with understanding, and when life becomes demanding
> Help us turn to you for strength to find our way.

> Join our hands, Father, as we
> Take each step ahead together. We pray for unity.

May we know the joy of giving; may we share the joys of living.
Until hand in hand we face eternity, help us live for Thee.

"There is no fear in love. But perfect love drives out fear . . ."
(1 John 4:18)

So many years you have been there
To love and cherish, honor, care.
But now it's time to lean on me.
Lord, help me be just what he needs.

Getting It Right...

Dear Vickiey
I love you
Zachary B.

These words were scribbled on a note pad by my nephew when he was six years old, and can still be found six years later under a magnet on my refrigerator. Just learning to write and spell, Zac had an important message for me and presumably wanted to be sure it was correct. Since my first name can be and frequently is spelled several different ways (ending in *i* or *ie* or *ey* or *y*), Zac apparently wasn't sure which letters he needed, so he just used them all . . . V-i-c-k-i-e-y. In doing so, he not only gave me a treasured remembrance of his childhood, but also unknowingly illustrated an important truth: When something is really important to us, we will do as much as we can to get it right.

"Getting it right" as a caregiver can be a challenge for several reasons. First, most family caregivers have little or no training in meeting the physical and emotional needs of the care recipient. Caregivers often have to actively pursue training on things as basic as proper lifting techniques to prevent injury to either party, not to mention more complex matters such as financial and legal issues. Caregivers should not hesitate to ask questions of health care providers, financial advisors, and attorneys until they have the information they need.

Another reason "getting it right" can become complicated for a caregiver is what I like to call "the changing landscape." Frequently, the conditions that create a need for caregiving in the first place may also result in inconsistency and volatility on the part of the care recipient. Involuntarily, the care recipient may perceive something as "right" one moment but "entirely wrong" the next. Keep in mind that irritating or seemingly vindictive behavior is often beyond the control of the person receiving care.

Finally, "getting it right" can be difficult when the caregiver fails to have empathy—to feel what the care recipient feels. "Try to put yourself in the patient's shoes. You will feel less angry the tenth time you are asked what day it is if you think about how it must be not to know when it is or where things are."[1]

For Jesus Christ, "getting it right" meant much more than walking in another person's shoes. Leaving the splendor of heaven, "the Word became flesh and dwelt among us." God literally *became man*, but He didn't stop there! Jesus lovingly and sacrificially *became sin* for us. "He made the One who did not know sin to be sin for us, so that we might become the righteousness of God in Him" (2 Corinthians 5:21 HCSB). Through His death on the cross, Jesus was able to defeat sin and death, cancel our sin debt, and become the bridge over the chasm that separated holy God and sinful humanity. Now that's what I call "getting it right"!

*"To reconcile everything to Himself through Him by mak-
ing peace through the blood of His cross. . . . He erased the
certificate of debt, with its obligations, that was against us
and opposed to us, and has taken it out of the way by nail-
ing it to the cross."*

(Colossians 1:20 and 2:14 HCSB)

I used to try with all my might
To follow rules, to do what's right.
But now I know that I am free
Because You paid it all for me.

Controlling Worry and Anxiety...

Most likely, you are familiar with the serenity prayer of St. Francis of Assisi:

God grant me the serenity to accept the things I cannot change,
The courage to change the things I can,
And the wisdom to know the difference.

In his prayer, St. Francis reminds us of the futility of worry. In essence, he tells us that it is useless to worry about things we *can* change. Rather than worrying, we should use our energy and time to accomplish change. In like manner, it makes no sense to worry about things we *cannot* change because no matter how much we worry, they're not going to change. Instead, we should channel our efforts in a more positive and productive direction.
 In caregiving, issues arise over which we have no control, but about which much time and energy can be wasted by

worrying. Often, these are "how long" questions: How long will I have my loved one with me? How long will our finances hold out? How long will I hold out? How long will my loved one remember me? How long until the condition worsens? While worries and fears are normal in caregiving, excessive anxiety can interfere with daily functioning and can even cause physical symptoms such as headaches, stomach upsets, rapid breathing, fast heart rate, trembling, and irritability.

"The key to managing anxiety is to find the balance between reality, fears, and worries. Stay focused on this balance, and do not give in to excessive negative thoughts," psychologist Dr. Shachi Shantinath tells caregivers. "Pay attention to your breathing when you feel anxious or fearful. Take deep, full, and slow breaths and that will help to return a sense of calm." Additionally, prayer and meditation are effective ways to still the mind when worries are rampant.[1]

Before St. Francis and before Dr. Shantinath, the apostle Paul identified the importance of prayer in controlling anxiety. In Philippians 4:6, Paul suggests that we replace our anxieties with prayer, our worries with thanksgiving, and our uncertainties with requests to God. Remember, life's worries will never knock you for a loop when you are leaning on the everlasting arms.

"Do not be anxious about anything, but in everything, by prayer and petition, with thanksgiving, present your requests to God."

(Philippians 4:6)

We are so prone to worry, Lord,
Instead of trusting in your Word,
The things we cannot change, You can
When we just place them in your hands.

Caring for the Terminally Ill . . .

Today I want to share with you a poem written by a friend of mine for her stepmother, who was the caregiver for her terminally ill father. I believe my friend, Sandra Winner, does a marvelous job of capturing the struggles and commitments of "The Caregiver's World."

I am watching the world, people rushing to and fro
Their minds are on their duties
My mind is full of memories

I used to be like them, one day I'll join their rank
But today I'm on the outside,
living with the dying
Consumed with the struggling of another

Once he was strong like I am, but now he is frail
each day seems slow with forced routine
but our trip is almost through as I watch him quickly
fail

I want to spend it wisely, this time will not last
Savoring each stolen quiet moment
Reminiscing, reliving, and sharing the past

It's hard to be where I am, My heart is filled with
grief
So many questions to be answered
But for him it's like relief

Do you see me as you hurry to and fro
Only the facade you want to see
I am beside you but not with you. Do you see me?

I long to join you from this place
I will not leave the struggles he must face
He brought me here through your rushing world
Now he needs my tending
to bring him through this time of ending

Someday I will not be consumed by him, My world
returned to me
But I will have my memories
of this time of ending and his time of strength.[1]

*"Entreat me not to leave thee, or to return from following
after thee: for whither thou goest, I will go; and where
thou lodgest, I will lodge; thy people shall be my people,
and thy God my God. Where thou diest, will I die, and*

there will I be buried: the Lord do so to me, and more also, if ought but death part me and thee."

(Ruth 1:16–17 KJV)

Lord, we know the end is near.
I know it; so does he.
Help us to face it without fear,
For we are safe in Thee.

Learning Lessons from a Cat...

If you are a cat person, you will undoubtedly relate to these caregiving lessons from the cat! If you're not a cat person, the following provide a good summary of key points from previous devotionals. Either way, here are some words of wisdom and advice from our furry friends:[1]

(1) *Take a happy nap on the couch.* Caregiving can be exhausting, so catch a little down time whenever you can.

(2) *Get petted as often as possible.* Caregivers need regular breaks from their routine responsibilities. Find ways to pamper yourself occasionally.

(3) *Land on your feet every time you fall.* Caregivers should seek to maintain balance in their lives. With balance, every small slip won't turn your world upside down.

(4) *Be aware when something's fishy.* Unfortunately, caregivers and their care recipients, especially senior adults, can be easy prey for dishonesty and

scams. The old saying is true: If it seems too good to be true, it probably is!

(5) *Stay on top of things.* Caregiving usually comes with medical, business, and financial issues to be handled. Don't procrastinate or ignore them.

(6) *Don't dig in the litter for very long.* Almost everyone experiences negative thoughts and self-pity at times, but don't allow yourself to dwell in them.

(7) *When you have a fur ball, cough it up.* Holding feelings and emotions inside can be unhealthy, both physically and emotionally. Let them out by sharing with a friend or support group.

(8) *Curiosity never killed anything except a little time.* Don't hesitate to ask lots of questions to those who help with medical, financial, and legal issues.

(9) *You can only stretch so far.* Be careful not to stretch yourself too thin. Be aware of when you are reaching your limits, and ask for help.

(10) *Scratch when it itches.* Taking care of your own needs as well as those of the care recipient will help prevent burnout.

(11) *Get someone else to clean your bathroom.* As a caregiver, don't try to go it alone. Ask others for assistance with everyday tasks while you carry out your caregiving responsibilities.

(12) *Always rest in the sun* . . . or in our case, the Son. In the midst of all the activities and responsibilities that accompany caregiving, find your rest in the Son, who issues this invitation: "Come to me, all you who are weary and burdened, and I will give you rest" (Matthew 11:28).

"But ask the animals, and they will teach you, or the birds of the air, and they will tell you; or speak to the earth, and it will teach you, or let the fish of the sea inform you. Which of all these does not know that the hand of the Lord has done this? In His hand is the life of every creature and the breath of all mankind."

(Job 12:7–10)

Teach me lessons everyday
From everything that comes my way.
Creation shows Your power, Lord,
In ways too mighty to ignore.

DAY 34

Relating to Others...

Whether we like to admit it or not, caregiving can impact not only the relationship between caregiver and care recipient, but also other relationships with family, friends, and co-workers. For instance, family members who see the loved one infrequently may think the caregiver exaggerates the extent of care needed. Out-of-town siblings may become critical of the care being given, question decisions made by the caregiver, or experience feelings of guilt for not being able to help more. These reactions can then cause the caregiver to feel resentful or unappreciated, resulting in strained family relationships.[1]

Friendships can also bear the brunt of caregiving stress. As mentioned previously, caregivers have a tendency to isolate themselves from friends and social situations for many reasons, not the least of which is lack of time and energy. Additionally, caregivers for those whose functioning has changed because of severe illness or injury report that friends sometimes seem uncomfortable with the new situation and, after the initial outpouring of concern, tend to drift away.[2]

In the work arena, caregiving responsibilities may affect the employer/employee relationship in a negative manner. "Employers might not recognize that they have an employee who comes to their job and works a full eight- or ten-hour day; then that same employee leaves work to go care for an elderly parent or loved one," says Brad Hancock of Paragon Senior Care. "Their day may not end until very late at night." While employers and co-workers are generally understanding of childcare problems, they may not understand eldercare needs. According to the National Family Caregivers Association, however, eldercare is projected to replace childcare as the number one dependent care issue in the United States by 2005.[3]

So what's a Christian caregiver to do in the face of potential relationship problems such as these? Consider the advice of the apostle Paul:

"Don't have anything to do with foolish and stupid arguments, because you know they produce quarrels. And the Lord's servant must not quarrel; instead he must be kind to everyone, able to teach, not resentful" (2 Timothy 2:23–24).

"And I want you to stress these things, so that those who have trusted in God may be careful to devote themselves to doing what is good. These things are excellent and profitable to everyone. But avoid foolish controversies and genealogies and arguments and quarrels . . . because these are unprofitable and useless" (Titus 2:8–9).

"Bear with one another and forgive whatever grievances you may have against one another. Forgive as the Lord forgave you. And over all these virtues put on love, which binds them all together in perfect unity" (Colossians 3:13–14).

"Live in harmony with one another. Do not be proud . . . . If it is possible, as far as it depends on you, live at peace with everyone. Do not be overcome by evil, but overcome evil with good" (Romans 12:16–18, 21). Enough said!

"Whatever happens, conduct yourselves in a manner worthy of the gospel of Christ."

(Philippians 1:27a)

Help us avoid the petty things
And quarrels they so easily bring.
Rather to live peaceably,
We look to you for unity.

Moving Beyond Good Intentions...

Caregiving can be filled with good intentions: *I'm going to be more patient with the one I'm caring for. I'm going to take better care of myself. I'm going to stop putting off that decision. I'm going to find time to start going to that support group. I'm going to ask _____ for a little help with _____.* (You fill in the blanks!) While it's important to make those kinds of decisions, moving beyond good intentions requires more than just deciding.

In his Christian counseling seminars, my brother adapts the story of six little frogs sitting on a log. One of the frogs says, "I'm going to jump off this log!" My brother then asks, "How many frogs are left on the log?" Most of the time the seminar participants respond, "Five." "No," my brother retorts, "there are still six, because the first frog never really got around to jumping!" His point, of course, is that deciding to do something, or even talking about doing something, is different than actually doing it.[1]

We human beings are experts at having good intentions. How many of us made New Year's resolutions this year, just to break them before February? How many diets or exercise programs have we begun, only to fall off the wagon? How many times have we said, "I'm going to get my taxes done early this year," and then find ourselves filling out tax forms at midnight on April 14? How many of you have read something in this book, decided to make a change, and like the little frog on the log, just haven't gotten around to it?

In Philippians, Paul says that God works in us "to will and to do." *To will* (deciding) is followed by *to do* (taking action). Choosing to take action on a decision is what moves us beyond good intentions. Perhaps Nike has the right idea when their ads encourage us, "Just Do It!"

As we near the end of *Forty Days of Care*, my prayer is that something you have read has triggered ideas about things you need to do or perhaps stop doing. More important than reading anything written in these pages, however, will be asking the same question Saul asked when he encountered Christ on the road to Damascus: "Lord, what wilt thou have me to do?" (Acts 22:10 KJV).

Ask yourself that question, listen for His answer, and then . . .

"*. . . do it, not only when their eye is on you and to win their favor, but with sincerity of heart and reverence for the Lord. Whatever you do, work at it with all your heart, as working for the Lord, not for men.*"

(Colossians 3:22–23)

Lord, You know I mean well when
I just resolve to do again
The things I've meant to do before . . .
Remind me who I'm working for.

Looking Up...

ast evening, my nephew and I went to a local sporting goods store to look for his new baseball shoes. Being a large warehouse-type store, it offered a huge selection of brands and styles. After spending quite a while deciding among the numerous options, we began to look for the right size. It seemed they had every size except the right one, as I dug through the boxes on the double-deep shelves in front of me. As my frustration was about to get the best of me, I placed my hands on my hips and took a deep breath. These actions caused my head to lift, and as I looked up, I saw stacks and stacks of boxes with shoes of all sizes stored on shelves above the display. I had been "spinning my wheels" looking all around me for what I needed, when all I had to do was look up!

We tend to make the same mistake with our emotional and spiritual needs. Whether coping with loneliness, emptiness, grief, guilt, or the many other feelings we encounter, our first reaction often is to look to people and things around us to meet our needs. Don't get me wrong: I truly believe that God provides friends, pastors, counselors, support groups and others to help us through the hard times, often serving as an extension of God's hands in the world. Nevertheless, it's important to remember that to find fully what we need, we've got to look up!

Consider an instance when Jesus looked up: ". . . and *looking up* to heaven, he blessed, and brake, and gave the loaves to his disciples, and the disciples to the multitude" (Matthew 14:19b KJV, EMPHASIS ADDED). Each of His actions in this verse has its own significance: *Looking up to heaven*, Jesus was acknowledging the Source of His power and provision. When *he blessed*, he demonstrated His reliance on the power of prayer. As He *brake* and *gave*, Jesus acted upon His prayer with faith. Finally, He *gave the loaves to his disciples and the disciples to the multitude*, depending on His followers as extensions of Himself to meet the needs of those who needed to be nourished and restored.

For caregivers, unresolved emotions can easily lead to burnout. Gerontologist Nancy Wexler states, "It is entirely understandable and human that any person who shoulders full responsibility for another should burn out. Caring for someone who cannot survive without you is both emotionally and physically draining, no matter how much you may love the person." [1] So when you are feeling especially human and when burnout is smoldering just below the surface, LOOK UP. As the psalmist expressed it, "I will lift up my eyes to the hills—where does my help come from? My help comes from the Lord, the Maker of heaven and earth" (Psalm 121:1–2). Restoration comes when we look up, acknowledge the Source of our strength, rely on the power of prayer, act upon our prayers in faith, and depend upon those God chooses to use as channels of His blessings in our lives.

"After that he put his hands again upon his eyes, and made him look up; and he was restored . . ."

(Mark 8:25 KJV)

We lift our eyes to You, our God,
For strength to walk each path we trod.
And when we feel we can't do more,
We look to You to be restored.

DAY 37

Overcoming Obstacles...

E ncountering and overcoming obstacles is a part of every aspect of our lives, and caregiving is no exception. In addition to medical and financial obstacles related to the loved one's condition, caregiving may also build walls of isolation, relationship problems, family stress, and emotional strain. Overcoming these kinds of obstacles is extremely important, but often difficult.

Joshua and the Israelites faced a huge obstacle soon after crossing the Jordan River to enter the Promised Land. Their obstacle, of course, was the wall around Jericho. We all know the story . . . if not from the Scriptures, then from the old spiritual song. And we know what happens: "Joshua fought the battle of Jericho, and the walls came tumbling down!" As we seek to overcome our own obstacles, perhaps we can learn a few strategies from Joshua:

(1) *Recognize the power and holiness of God.* Before Joshua received God's message about Jericho, he

was told to remove his sandals because he was on holy ground. He did so without hesitation.

(2) *Listen to the Lord's instructions and follow them.* God's plan for overcoming the obstacle at Jericho may have seemed a little strange to Joshua, but he followed it exactly as he was told.

(3) *Rely on the spiritual leaders God has placed in your life.* After receiving God's directions, Joshua relayed the message to the Israelites. When Joshua had spoken to the people, he ordered them, "Advance!" and they did.

(4) *Trust the Lord's timing.* God commanded Joshua and the army of Israel to march around the city of Jericho for six days and then on the seventh day to march around it seven times. Only then was God ready to give them the city. Acting too quickly or waiting too long undoubtedly would have brought disaster.

(5) *Remember God can provide a way out in the midst of chaos.* Inside Jericho, Rahab and her family seemed destined for annihilation as were the other residents of the city. However, God—and therefore Joshua—did not forget her.

(6) *Give the Lord what belongs to Him.* Joshua told his soldiers, "All the silver and gold and the articles of bronze and iron are sacred to the Lord and must go into his treasury." (Joshua 6:19)

(7) *Believe that God can overcome obstacles that seem insurmountable.* Facing a massive walled city that was "tightly shut up," Joshua and the Israelites believed the word of the Lord . . . and the walls came tumbling down!

"The seventh time around, when the priests sounded the trumpet blast, Joshua commanded the people, 'Shout! For the Lord has given you the city!' . . . and at the sound of the trumpet, when the people gave a loud shout, the wall collapsed . . ."

(Joshua 6:16, 20)

Facing walls and obstacles
We cannot climb alone,
We lift our voices up to You,
For You can bring them down.

Improving as a Caregiver...

As I worked on this project, I kept several folders on my computer desktop for devotionals in various stages of completion. I had entitled one folder "caregiver in progress" for pieces I had just started or ideas for new ones. I looked at that folder many, many times before I realized that's what I was . . . a caregiver in progress. Do you remember the children's song, "He's Still Working on Me" or the bumper sticker that read, "Be patient. God's not finished with me yet"? That's me as a caregiver! As I researched and wrote these daily readings, I often found myself thinking, "Do as I say, not as I do," knowing I still had a long way to go before I was really following my own advice. But that's okay, because caregiving—like child rearing—doesn't come with instructions . . . or does it?

Thankfully, there are many resources available to those who need help or information. These are a few of the numerous books available:

- *And Thou Shalt Honor: The Caregiver's Companion* (McLeod, ed.)
- *The Comfort of Home: An Illustrated Step-by-Step Guide* (Meyer)
- *The Complete Guide To Eldercare* (Jones-Lee and Callender)
- *The Fearless Caregiver* (Barg)
- *Fourteen Friends Guide to Eldercaring* (Cooper, ed.)
- *The Gift of Caregiving* (Goldman)
- *How To Care for Aging Parents: A Complete Guide* (Morris)
- *I'll Take Care of You* (Ilardo and Rothman)

Additionally, the "dot.com" world provides a plethora of information sources for the internet user. Here are just a few: www.aarp.org, www.aoa.dhhs.gov, www.caregiver.org, www.caregiver.com, www.caregiving.com, www.caregiving.org, www.careguide.net, www.eldercare.gov, and www.nfcacares.org.

All of these are great resources, but none can compare to the very best instruction book of all—the Holy Bible. In its pages, God has given us the instruction book for every aspect of life. As I hope I've demonstrated in these readings, all the joys, sorrows, rewards, and frustrations of caregiving are addressed more than adequately in the Scriptures. His Word gives us instructions on how to mature as Christians and how to develop Christlike character. As Rick Warren reminds us, "There is only one way to develop the habits of Christlike character: You must *practice* them—and that takes time! *There are no instant habits.* Paul urged Timothy, '*Practice these things. Devote your life to them so that everyone can see your progress*'" (1 Timothy 4:15 GWT).[1] As we allow the Holy Spirit to produce the fruit of love, joy, peace, patience, gentleness, goodness, meekness, self-control and faith in our lives, and as we practice Christlike character daily, we can improve not only in our caregiving, but in all we do.

> *"Being confident of this, that he who began a good work in you will carry it on to completion until the day of Christ Jesus."*
>
> (Philippians 1:6)

I know I'm not all I should be
Or everything You want for me.
Lord, make me just a ball of clay
So you can mold me in Your way.

Saying Goodbye...

If the Lord tarries, most of us will come to the point of saying goodbye to the loved one for whom we have provided care and support. For some, the journey to that place will be long and difficult. Others will feel helpless as the time speeds by uncontrollably fast. How should we approach the process of saying goodbye? The answer was brought into focus for me by an article in *Baylor Magazine*, which I cut out and hung near my mirror so that I would see it everyday.

In the article, Dr. Lauren Barron, a physician in private practice in Waco, Texas, tells of a lesson she learned while in medical school. A lecturer on Alzheimer's explained to the med students that he and his wife cared for a dear relative who could not walk, talk, bathe, or clothe herself. She was in diapers and required constant supervision, yet the speaker spoke with delight of the pleasure and privilege of caring for her. Then he revealed he was talking about their infant daughter, not an elderly relative as the students assumed.

"I never have forgotten his point about how gladly we care for our babies—how tenderly and lovingly and with what joy and hope. But *the same care* required by our elders, we give grudgingly, with pity or dread and with a sense of futility, tragedy, and grief," Dr. Barron states. "He challenged us to approach the care of the elderly, whether as physicians or family members, with more hope, more optimism, more joy and more of a sense of privilege—to say goodbye as well as we say hello."[1]

As caregivers, we do not control when or where we will say goodbye to our loved one. What we can control is *how*—our attitudes and actions during the process of saying goodbye. Whether that process is long or short, it matters how we treat those whose care God has entrusted to us. It matters that we say goodbye with love and kindness and, yes, even with joy.

"And this is my prayer: that your love may abound more and more in knowledge and depth of insight so that you may be able to discern what is best . . ."
(Philippians 1:9–10a)

Lord, you know that we will cry
When it's time to say goodbye,
But may we trust our last farewell
Means they're home with You to dwell.

Saying Hello Again...

As I write today, little signs of spring have begun to show themselves. Trees are beginning to bud; flowers are starting to blossom; birds are singing happily in the backyard. All around me the things that looked so desolate during the dead of winter show signs of new life. In all of nature, spring reminds us that death is not the end. On the contrary, it is the beginning of new life. For Christians, death is "to be absent from the body and to be present with Christ," who guides us as we take our next step into eternity (2 Corinthians 5:8 KJV).

Caregiving often ends with the care recipient making the transition from the arms of the caregiver into the arms of the Lord. While saying goodbye will naturally bring sorrow, we as Christians can be comforted in the fact that our goodbyes are not forever.

As we complete our forty days together, I want to leave you with several thoughts of comfort and assurance. Whether your goodbyes are close at hand, far into the future, or already spoken, the Lord wants to remind you that you will be saying "hello" again!

First, Jesus has already won the victory over death. "Death has been swallowed up in victory. O death, where is thy sting? O grave, where is thy victory? . . . But thanks be to God, which giveth us the victory through our Lord Jesus Christ" (1 Corinthians 15:54–55, 57 KJV).

Next, Jesus promised He is preparing a place for us. "In my Father's house are many rooms; if it were not so, I would have told you. I am going there to prepare a place for you. And if I go and prepare a place for you, I will come back and take you with me that you also may be where I am" (John 14:2–3).

In the meantime, Jesus leaves for us a supernatural peace. "Peace I leave with you; my peace I give you. I do not give to you as the world gives. Do not let your hearts be troubled, and do not be afraid" (John 14:27).

Finally, as Christians we will experience the eternal joys of heaven together. "And God shall wipe away every tear from their eyes; there shall be no more death, nor sorrow, nor crying. There shall be no more pain, for the former things have passed away" (Revelation 21:4 KJV).

". . . and so shall we ever be with the Lord. Wherefore, comfort one another with these words."

(1 Thessalonians 4:17–18 KJV)

Thank you for these words to share
With others as we seek to care.
Our joys and tears we'll bring to You
Until You have made all things new.
Amen.

Caregiver's Self-Rating Scale*

1. Abandonment—To withdraw protection or support or to actively abuse your care-receiver.
2. Neglect—To allow life-threatening situations to persist or to display consistent coldness or anger.
3. Detachment/aloofness—To maintain an air of detachment or being aloof, perfunctory in your care, no genuine concern, only obligation. Concerned only with the physical well-being of your care-receiver.
4. General support—Given freely, with a guarded degree of warmth and respect, occasional feeling of manipulation. Concerned with both emotional and physical well-being of care-receiver.
5. Express empathy—the ability to feel what your care-receiver feels, a quality relationship where feeling can be freely expressed and caringly received with non-judgmental positive regard.

6. Sympathy—Feeling sorry for the care-receiver, giving sympathy, focusing on the losses experienced by care-receiver.
7. Occasional over-involvement—Care characterized by periodic attempts to do for rather than be with.
8. Consistent over-involvement—Care-receiver regarded as object of series of tasks which must be performed.
9. Heroic over-involvement—Care characterized by sometimes frantic and desperate attempts to provide for every possible need your care-receiver has; increased dependence, care-receiver not allowed independence.
10. Fusion of personalities—Between caregiver and care-receiver. The caregiver's needs no longer have any value or meaning; the caregiver has abandoned herself to needs of the care-receiver.

---

*Used by permission from the San Diego Mental Health Services

End Notes

Introduction

(1)   "Family Caregiving Statistics." National Family Caregivers Association Website. <www.nfcacares. org/NFC2002_stats.html>, pp. 1–2.

(2)   Libert, Anne Blanford. "Elderly Parents and Adult Children as Caregivers. Highlights: An ERIC/CAPS Digest." ERIC Clearinghouse on Counseling and Personnel Services. ERIC Identifier: ED279993, p. 1.

(3)   "Taking Care of Others: Caregiving." Erie County Department of Senior Services Website. <www.erie.gov/depts/seniorservices/ taking_care_of_others.phtml>, p. 1.

(4)   "What Is Caregiving and Who Are America's Caregivers." National Family Caregivers Association Website. <www.nfcacares.org>, p. 1.

(5)   Warren, Rick. *The Purpose-Driven Life*. Grand Rapids, Michigan: Zondervan, 2002, pp. 9–10.

Day One

[1] "Brain Attack: The Family's Role in Caregiving." Dallas: American Heart Association Brochure, p. 22.

[2] "Elder Care." *PacifiCare Behavioral Health, Inc.* Website. <www.pbhi.com/members_public/ memyfamily/eldercare>, p. 1.

[3] "Caregiving: Managing Stress When Giving Care." *AARP Webplace.* <www.aarp.org/confacts/ caregive/mngstress>, pp. 1–5.

Day Three

[1] "Taking Care of Others," p.1.

[2] Calkin, Ruth Harms. *Tell Me Again, Lord, I Forget.* Colorado Springs, Colorado: David C. Cook Publishing Company, 1974.

Day Four

[1] "Looking Good Means Feeling Good." *CareGuide* Website. <www.careguide.com/Careguide/ healthwellbeing>, p. 1.

Day Five

[1] *Taylor Gifts Catalog 2003*, p. 63.

[2] "10 Timely Tips for Caregivers." *Senior Health Care* Website. <www.senior-health-care.com/ tips-for-caregivers.htm>, p. 1.

[3] "The Importance of Touch." *Aribella* Magazine Website. <www.aribella.com/touch.htm>, p. 1.

[4] "10 Timely Tips," p. 2.

Day Six

[1] Angelou, Maya. Hallmark's Maya Angelou Life Mosaic Collection. © 2003 Maya Angelou. Used by permission.

Day Seven

[1] Crawford, Dan R. *DiscipleShape: Twelve Weeks to Spiritual Fitness.* Peabody, MA: Hendrickson Publishers, 1998, pp. 94–96.

[2] "Alzheimer's Disease: What it is . . . What We're Doing About It!" Alzheimer's Disease and Related Disorders Association Pamphlet, 2003, p. 4.

[3] Crawford, p. 96.

Day Eight

[1] Sweat, Rebecca. "How Pets Help Senior Citizens." PetPlace.com Website. <www.petplace.netscape.com/articles>, p. 1.

[2] "The Healing Power of Pets." Pets and Senior Citizens Website. <www.seniors-site.com/petsm/needpets>, pp. 1–2.

[3] Wohlberg, Steve. *Will My Pet Go To Heaven?* Enumclaw, WA: WinePress Publishing, 2002.

Day Nine

[1] "Caregiving: Managing Stress," p. 3.

[2] Hunt, Dee Dee. "Caregiving." *Scleroderma from A to Z.* The International Scleroderma Network Website. <*www.sclero.org/support/ caregivers/dee-dee*>, p. 3.

(3) Brown, Denise M. "Focus on You: Tips for
     Caregivers." *Caregiving Newsletter Online Support
     August 1997*, <www.caregiving.com/support >, p. 4.
(4) From "Love Is Something You Do" by David Baker
     © 1969 Hope Publishing Co., Carol Stream, IL. All
     right reserved. Used by permission.
(5) "Christians, Anger, and Forgiveness." *Walking
     Wounded.Net* Website. <www.walking-wounded.net
     /html/anger.html>, pp. 4–5.

Day Eleven

(1) "UK: Care of the Elderly Often Lacks Dignity." Glo-
     bal Action on Aging Website. <www.globalaging.org
     /health/world/dignity>, May 28, 2003, p. 1.

Day Twelve

(1) Wooten, Patty. "Laughter as Therapy for Patient and
     Caregiver." *Pulmonary Rehabilitation*, ed. Hodgkin.
     Philadelphia: Lippincott, 1993.
(2) "Caring for the Caregiver." *The Caregiver's Hand-
     book*. San Diego County Mental Health Services.
     <www.acsu.buffalo.edu/~drstall/hndbk0.html>.

Day Thirteen

(1) Pfeiffer, Beverly. "Myths About the Aging Pro-
     cess." *Work and Family Life Newsletter*, October,
     1993, University of Missouri Outreach and Ex-
     tension. Available online at <www.outreach.
     missouri.edu/cmregion/thriving>.

[2] Abel, Barbara. "With Alzheimer's, the Caregiver Is a Patient, Too." *Healthlink* . Medical College of Wisconsin, 2003. Available online at <healthlink.mcw.edu/article/1031002313>.

[3] Neukrug, Linda. "October 27 Devotional." *Daily Guideposts 2001.* Carmel, NY: Guidepost, p. 314.

Day Fourteen

[1] "Alzheimer's Disease/Senility." Calgary Health Region Website. <www.calgaryhealthregion.ca/hlthconn/items/alz.htm>, p. 2.

Day Fifteen

[1] "In the Middle: A Report on Multicultural Boomers Coping with Family and Aging Issues." American Association of Retired Persons (AARP) Website. <www.aarp.org/inthemiddle>, pp. 1–2.

Day Sixteen

[1] "Alzheimer's Disease: What It Is . . . What We're Doing About It!" Alzheimer's Disease and Related Disorders Association Pamphlet, 2003, p. 4.

Day Seventeen

[1] Vieregg, Brenda Jones. "Exploring Eldercare." *News Hour with Jim Lehrer Transcript,* December 24, 1999. Available online on PBS Website <www.pbs.org/newshour/bb/health/july-dec99/eldercare>.

(2) Landy, Karen and Buettner, Linda. "Communicating with Your Care Receiver." *The Caregiver Manual and Caregiver Guide for Southwest Florida.* Florida Gulf Coast University Website. <www.fgcu.edu/cfpa/manual>.

Day Nineteen

(1) Adapted by permission from a speech given by Catherine Davis, February 28, 2004, Delta Kappa Gamma Area X Luncheon, Fort Worth, Texas.

Day Twenty

(1) Crawford, p. 24.

Day Twenty-Two

(1) Author Unknown.

Day Twenty-Three

(1) Brzowsky, Sara. "How To Be Stress-Resilient." *Parade Sunday Newspaper Magazine,* October 12, 2003, p. 12.

Day Twenty-Four

(1) Crawford, Dan R. *Night of Tragedy, Dawning of Light.* Colorado Springs, Colorado: Shaw Books, 2000, cover.

(2) Davis, Verdell. *Let Me Grieve But Not Forever.* Dallas: Word Publishing, 1994, p. 4.

Day Twenty-Five

(1) Banks, Carolyn. "Aging in Place Means Independence." *LifeTimes*, Blue Cross and Blue Shield of Texas Newsletter, January, 2004, p. 12.

(2) Banks, p. 12.

Day Twenty-Six

(1) Stanphill, Ira. "I Know Who Holds Tomorrow." Copyright 1950 by Ira Stanphill.

Day Twenty-Seven

(1) Russell, Bob and Scott, Bobby. "He Ain't Heavy; He's My Brother." Published by Hollies Music, 1970.

(2) Pek-san Lui and Nancy Martland. "Family Support: Siblings with Disabilities." Available online at <www.tufts.edu/cfn/family-storystarter/fs-siblingswithdisabilities.shtml>, pp. 1, 4.

Day Twenty-Eight

(1) Wexler, Nancy. "To Those Who Have Assumed the Role of Care-Giver." *Getting It Right* Newsletter, Issue 10, September, 2001. Available online at <www.nancy-wexler.com>.

Day Twenty-Nine

(1) The Well Spouse Foundation Website. <www.wellspouse.org>.

(2) "Caregiving for Spouses." Evergreen Commons Website. <www.evergreencommons.org>.

(3) "Alone Is Not Lonely." *Mainstay*, The Well Spouse Foundation Website. <www.wellspouse.org>.

[4]   Abel, pp. 1–2.

Day Thirty

[1]   "Tips for Family Caregivers." Erie County Department of Senior Services Website. <www.erie.gov/
depts/seniorservices/ TakeCareofYourself>, p. 1.

Day Thirty-One

[1]   Shantinath, Shachi D. "What to Do When You Feel
Scared, Anxious or Excessively Worried."
Caregivers' Center Website. <www.healthandage.
com, 2003.

Day Thirty-Two

[1]   Poem written by Sandra Winner, Fort Worth, Texas,
for Sandra S. Webb on November 8, 1998. Used by
permission.

Day Thirty-Three

[1]   Loosely based on "All I Need To Know, I Learned
from My Cat" by Suzy Becker.

Day Thirty-Four

[1]   Abel, Barbara, p. 2.
[2]   "Mainstay Forum—Coping." *Mainstay*, The Well
Spouse Foundation Website <www.wellspouse.org>,
p. 1.
[3]   "The New National Concern: Eldercare." *Spring
Lawn and Garden*, The Star Group, March 2004,
p. 3.

Day Thirty-Five

[1] Gilliam, Larry. "Experience Reparenting: A Re-opportunity To Have A Happy Childhood" (Seminar presented in Irving, Texas, 2004).

Day Thirty-Six

[1] Wexler, Nancy, p. 1.

Day Thirty-Eight

[1] Taken from PURPOSE-DRIVEN® LIFE, THE by Rick Warren. Copyright © 2002 by Rick Warren. Used by permission of The Zondervan Corporation.

Day Thirty-Nine

[1] Barron, Lauren. "There's Much To Learn in How We Say Goodbye." *Baylor Magazine*, March/April, 2003, p. 52. Used by permission of Baylor Magazine.

To order additional copies of

Forty Days of Care for the Caregiver

Have your credit card ready and call:

1-877-421-READ (7323)

or please visit our web site at
www.pleasantword.com

Also available at:
www.amazon.com
and
www.barnesandnoble.com

Printed in the United States
22993LVS00002B/382-405

9 781414 102030